Miracle Heidi

When Doctors Couldn't...
God Could!

by

Vickie Boone Watson

Sterling Press International
Bedford, Texas

Scripture quotations from:

Those marked KJV are from *The King James Version of the Bible.*

Those marked NIV are from *The Holy Bible, New International Version.* Copyright © 1973, 1978, 1984 International Bible Society.

Those marked NASB are from *The Ryrie Study Bible, New American Standard Translation.* Copyright © 1976, 1978 by The Moody Bible Institute of Chicago.

Miracle Heidi: When Doctors Couldn't . . . God Could!

Copyright © 1996 by Vickie Boone Watson

ISBN 0-9654974-0-2

Cover design and page layout by Jeff Wollman

Editing by Lena Dooley

Printed in the United States of America by Eerdman's Printing Company, Grand Rapids, Michigan

"That I may publish with the voice

of thanksgiving,

and tell of all thy wondrous works."

(Psalm 26:7, KJV)

To the Glory of God

ACKNOWLEDGMENTS

Thank you to my dear husband, Chuck. You believed in me. You believed in this project. And you sacrificed to make it happen. Thank you for vacation days spent feeding, diapering, loving, and playing with three, then four, little ones. For patience with a raging-hormones, pregnant writer. For keen business skills that brought the manuscript through the publication stage. For being a wonderful life companion. Life with you has never been boring!

Thank you to Sterling, Heidi, Holly, and Landon. You enrich my life daily. Each time I came out of seclusion in the upstairs office, your welcoming hugs and kisses reassured me of your love. You are special and a blessing.

Thank you to our parents, Algie and Ruth Boone of McComb, Mississippi, and Sarah Watson of Tipp City, Ohio. You placed your lives on hold for many long weeks to fight the battle with us at Heidi's bedside. We are grateful for your sacrificial love.

Thank you to Rebecca Laird, a dear friend and gifted writer. Our late-night, long distance conversations in the beginning days of this project taught me more about writing than any college course ever could.

Thank you to Rev. Travis Hutchison (theological consultant) and Dr. Robert Mann (medical consultant) for reviewing the manuscript for accuracy.

Thank you to the hundreds of friends and family members who walked with us through these days. Your love, prayers, and helping hands have blessed our lives. May God return that blessing to you.

Contents

FOREWORD

I believe in healing and in miracles. I believe God is present in all healing whether it is by a surgeon's hand or a supernatural touch from God. As Heidi's pediatrician, I saw a newborn baby who was very sick, and for the first month her condition went downhill daily. The only thing that could save her would be a miracle.

I don't use the word lightly, but Heidi's healing *was* through the miraculous touch of Jesus. If a physician were to give her a routine physical today, he would find a normal healthy child. It would be difficult, if not impossible, to detect the battle that occurred within her body.

This book chronicles the true story of Heidi's journey, as well as Vickie's struggles as the mother of an extremely sick child. The depths of the spiritual insights may challenge you as they did me. I had never seen God work in exactly this way before.

And there are other miracles in the Watson family history: the story of a thirty-six-year-old bachelor who many of us thought would never marry; the merging of two opposites into a delightful team; Chuck's and Vickie's decision to start a family at the age when most adults are finishing theirs — but perhaps that will be Vickie's next book!

It is a joy to be this family's doctor. I trust that you will be blessed and encouraged as you read this inspirational story of God's power and mercy.

Robert W. Mann, M.D., F.A.A.P.
Physicians Resource Council, Focus on the Family

Introduction

God miraculously healed our baby. This is a story of healing, but equally a story of my journey of faith as a mother.

It was not an instant McDonald's® drive-through version of a miracle—it was a painstakingly long, painful process. Neither was ours the experience of a "name it and claim it" gospel. No, it was a matter of hearing what *God* wanted for the situation and holding on to His Word regardless of what our eyes saw.

I understand less today about the how and the why of healing. Yet I understand more about the mercy and power of God. He was true to *every* word He spoke to us during those months. He supplied the needs of our family in every arena of life.

Please keep in mind two foundational premises as you read Heidi's story —

(1) I am not against the medical community. We had some of the finest doctors and nurses in the world, and we are grateful for their care. But I am thankful that we were not limited to their abilities.

(2) There are many who have prayed and stood firmly, believing for the healing of a loved one, just as we did. But your story ended differently. My purpose is not to heap more pain or guilt onto an already painful situation. I will *not* tell you that had you done certain things, your loved one would be healed or alive today. God does not work in that way. He is a loving and merciful God whose ways are far beyond ours.

I still have many burning questions for Him about healing. So watch for me—I'll be the one holding a list of questions, waiting in line at the pearly gates, with you.

Chapter One

FEARFULLY AND WONDERFULLY MADE

It was 2:26 p.m. on a cold Thursday afternoon in November. But I was sweating from labor—the kind that births babies.

Dr. Guthrie had just placed a bloody squirming little body on my stomach with the pronouncement, "It's a girl."

Her feeble attempts to cry only produced squeaks. Her skin was blue. I knew that wasn't normal.

"Take her," I pleaded. "Something's wrong." Hours later I felt guilty that those were my welcoming words to my little girl. It was a plea for help. I hoped she sensed that.

My husband Chuck cut the umbilical cord.

Nurse Nancy stood to my left gently crooning, "Come on. Come on." After a few seconds she glanced nervously toward the doctor at the foot of my bed.

The nursery nurse commanded, "Give her a minute."

I handed the baby back to Dr. Guthrie. "Get your motor started," he encouraged as he quickly passed her to the nursery team. "The cord was wrapped around her neck."

After a few more split-second cries, the nursery nurse announced, "Do you hear her crying? She's okay."

Nurse Nancy continued to croon, "Come on. Come on," as her eyes darted back and forth uneasily between the baby and Dr. Guthrie.

Seconds later the nursery nurse pushed the intercom button and commanded, "Yes, we need Cammie over here STAT!"

Within minutes, there were four people working on her. Alarms sounded from her bed as she continued to try to cry in split-second bursts of unnatural sound. Between each attempted cry, there was silence except for the alarms indicating that she was not breathing.

Chuck made a frantic call from my bedside to the church office—"It's a girl. She's having trouble breathing. Pray!"

Dr. Guthrie's attention had focused back on me. Still on supplemental oxygen. Body shaking uncontrollably. Temperature of 102. Plummeting blood pressure. What was wrong?

Chuck stood at my side, helplessly watching first me, then our blue baby girl struggling on her little bed only three feet away. His heart cried out to God as the fear rose within him that he might lose us both.

My sporadic thoughts? Denial. This had to be a mistake. It could not be happening—not after the promises from God during my pregnancy. He had sent several powerful messages to me about this baby. And not after the illness of our first child. You don't birth two sick babies. It just doesn't happen. Somebody wake me! This has to be a nightmare!

On another Thursday afternoon, only eight months earlier, Chuck and I had sat in an empty waiting room looking like most weary parents of a sick infant. Outdoors the month of March had brought an early spring to the Dallas/Fort Worth area. Hopefully the warmer weather would bring us a reprieve after the long winter. Four months of ear infections, respiratory viruses, croup, and surgery for ear tubes had worn us down.

Dr. Mann, our pediatrician, sent us to the x-ray lab across the lane from his office. He wanted Sterling's lungs x-rayed. This appeared to be a major asthma attack, possibly headed toward pneumonia. We squirmed in our chairs as Sterling's cries rang down the hall from the lab.

From that first cry at his birth fourteen months earlier, Sterling David Watson had wrapped his fingers around our hearts. We were ready for the adventure of parenting.

Oh, there had been plenty of adventure in our lives during our first six and one-half years of marriage "B.C."—before children. In an average year, approximately six hundred people passed through our home—for dinner, overnight stays, dessert, or a cup of tea. It was the ministry God had given us, that of hospitality. And we enjoyed it. It was always exciting to see who He brought across our path. This had also opened the door for us to share about hospitality in seminars and retreats.

We had spent exciting vacations volunteering in different parts of the world, thanks to Chuck's job in the training department of American Airlines. One Thanksgiving we delivered turkeys to a Bible college in Switzerland. We smuggled Bibles into the former Soviet Union and met with underground church members. On another trip we volunteered at Mother Teresa's home for abandoned children in Calcutta, India. And Chuck made thirty-six trips to Haiti (two trips since I joined the picture) to deliver donated medicine. That's what we did in our "spare" time apart from our jobs in the airline industry (Chuck) and mortgage banking (me).

These had also been exciting years of spiritual growth as we worked as laymen in planting a new church. Chuck now worked part-time there as business administrator. We were definitely not bored. Life was fulfilling.

Then a new season entered our lives—"Parenting 101." At thirty-five, I exchanged my wool business suits for denim and came home to suburban Bedford, Texas, nestled between Dallas and Fort Worth, to be a stay-at-home mom. Life had been full the past fourteen months since

Sterling's birth.

My mind played a fast forward video of those months as new parents. The first three had been a blur of sleepless nights, hours of painful screaming (Sterling, not me, although I often wanted to), and medical testing to find out if something was wrong with this child or if we were "weakling" parents.

"All babies cry . . . It's your first, you know, and you'll get used to it after awhile . . . our baby had colic, too." I hated those words which often came our way from seasoned, well-meaning parents.

But something just hadn't seemed right. Yes, babies do cry—but thirteen out of sixteen hours? Yes, they like to be held—but why would he wake up screaming within minutes of being laid in his cradle?

Finally when he was three months old, we received a diagnosis—reflux esophagitis—a condition where the muscle between the esophagus and stomach does not close after eating. This causes the contents of the stomach to back up into the esophagus, bathing it in acid. That explained the hours of holding him upright and finally laying a sleeping child flat in the cradle, only to have him screaming minutes later. Gravity was not in our favor if we wanted this child in his bed.

So for months we piled pillows under Chuck's head, and he slept in a near-upright position with Sterling on his chest. Sterling wanted to nurse every time we placed him on my chest, so this became a nightly father and son time of mega-bonding. By the time he was six months old, the medicines were starting to control the acid much of the time. And just two weeks ago, we had been able to discontinue his medication. End of reflux chapter.

Beginning of asthma chapter. How I hated that word!

The "stop" button clicked on my mental video and my thoughts returned to the present, to the quietness in the x-ray waiting room. How could I share with Chuck my news from that morning? Given the way the afternoon was going, my idea of a candle-light dinner appeared to be fading.

As we waited for the x-ray technician to bring Sterling back to us, Chuck solved my dilemma. "Vickie, I know we want another child, but at times like this I wonder how we could handle two. The stress of Sterling's medical problems has drained both of us. I just don't know how we would do it," he confided.

Linking my arm through his, I leaned across the arm rests between us and smiled demurely. "I think we'd better figure it out quickly."

He slowly turned his face toward me and, seeing my sheepish grin, turned in his chair to face me. "Are we—are you trying to tell me something? Wait a minute. You never told me what your doctor said this morning. Are we pregnant?" he questioned.

"Yes, baby Watson number two is on the way! Can you believe it? I feel so blessed." As we hugged there in the empty waiting room, I was once again awed by the miracle of conception—the same as with our first pregnancy. Yes, we both understood biology. But conception and birth were so amazing. Absolute miracles! How could anyone witness the birth of a baby and not believe in God?

Chuck had already forgotten the concerns he voiced only a minute earlier. He got as excited about our pregnancy as I did. This man was always full of surprises. On our wedding day, almost seven years earlier, I had thanked God for saving a thirty-six year old, never-married, godly man for me. I had been assured by the skeptics that what I was waiting for did not exist. And yet there he was at my side—a wonderful mixture of corporate skills, godly wisdom, faithful husband, and A-1 father all rolled into one handsome package. He stood six feet tall with thick red hair sprinkled with much more gray over the past year.

We were quickly brought back to focus on baby Watson number one as the technician returned a whimpering Sterling to us. His breathing was labored, the wheezing evident with each breath. We had a sick little boy. Hadn't he been through enough already?

We walked back across the shady lane, x-rays in hand, to Dr. Mann's office. Bob Mann had been a faithful encourager throughout Sterling's illness. He was a dear friend and an experienced pediatrician who had never given us the "all babies cry" speech. What an unbeatable combination! The first five words out of Bob's mouth let us know that he anticipated our first question. "If this were my child, I would hospitalize him. He needs continual breathing treatments under a mist tent for at least one night. Why don't we try this and see how he's doing in the morning?" It was easy to trust his advice.

We headed straight to Arlington Memorial Hospital for our first overnight experience in the hospital with a little one. That night Chuck slept under the tent with Sterling. It seemed to be the easiest way to keep him calm and inside the tent. I lay at the foot of the large baby bed on a sofa, one of those "comfortable" blue vinyl hospital versions of a sofa/bed. Chuck's job—to keep Sterling inside the tent and sleeping as much as possible. My job—to get whatever they needed—diapers, bottles, drinks.

Between the sound of the breathing machine and Sterling's need for rest, we didn't talk much throughout the evening and night. So I had plenty of time for my own thoughts. Many times I smiled in the darkness as I lay there praying for the new life within me.

The next morning as we headed home from the hospital, I took with me my newly-developed "theology of childbirth." Baby number two represented a brand new chapter for the Watsons. This baby would be healthy from day one. After all, God would not give me two sick babies. He just wouldn't. And a healthy newborn would seem easy compared to our experiences of the past year. It was pay day for Vickie. I deserved this.

In the months ahead as we shared our good news with friends, they reinforced my thoughts. "You won't believe what it's like to bring a new-born home from the hospital who sleeps the majority of the time. Your children will only be twenty-one months apart, but you won't have to deal with the illness and doctor visits you've had. This will be good for both of you."

During those months, I waited expectantly for the scripture and the song which I had asked the Lord to give me for this child. That had been a special part of my pregnancy with Sterling, so I was excited to hear what He would say about this child.

I didn't have to wait long. On a beautiful spring morning in April, just three months into my pregnancy, I sensed the Holy Spirit's gentle nudge as I read Psalm 139. He kept bringing me back to verses thirteen through sixteen:

> *For Thou didst form my inward parts;*
> *Thou didst weave me in my mother's womb.*
> *I will give thanks to Thee, for I am fearfully and wonderfully made;*
> *Wonderful are Thy works, And my soul knows it very well.*
> *My frame was not hidden from Thee, When I was made in secret,*
> *And skillfully wrought in the depths of the earth.*
> *Thine eyes have seen my unformed substance;*
> *And in Thy book they were all written,*
> *The days that were ordained for me,*
> *When as yet there was not one of them.*
>
> (Psalm 139:13-16, NASB)

"Are you sure, God?" I questioned. "I mean, this is beautiful. And it's powerful. But it's such a *normal* verse for a baby. Thousands of mothers have claimed this for the child in their womb. I wanted something unique." But the nudge did not go away. So I underlined the verses in my

Bible and noted in the margin "Baby Watson #2, 4/29/91." Oh well, maybe a better verse would come along later. Or maybe the baby's song would be more unusual.

By mid-August I was entering the last trimester of pregnancy. It was "nesting" time. Watch out! If you've ever experienced nesting instincts or lived with someone in the midst of nesting, you understand. Everything in the house got organized, thrown away, given away or carted away in a garage sale. Chuck accused me of getting rid of more than I kept. The "organizer" part of him loved it, but the "we-may-need-this-someday" part of him dreaded coming home each day to the line-up of large black trash bags. Closets, garage, attic room, nothing escaped my eye. Even the phone books under our bed were stacked by city—Fort Worth, Dallas, and mid-cities area. We had ten telephone books for the metropolitan area!

One Friday morning that August, still dressed in my nightgown, I had already been "nesting" for several hours. I stopped long enough to admire the fruit of my labor. The triple-sectioned wooden bookcase in our bedroom looked much better. With forty fewer books lining its shelves, I knew I would lie in bed tonight admiring its orderliness. One shelf now displayed framed family photos. Another held a few travel books and a copper airplane suspended from the shelf above.

It was almost ten o'clock, and any moment Sterling would be awakening from his morning nap upstairs. Hopefully there would be enough time for a bath and getting dressed before the sweet eighteen-month-old sound of "mama" came drifting down the stairs.

While waiting for the bathtub to fill, I turned on a local Christian radio station and heard Dr. James Dobson introducing his program for the day. He was re-playing a recording from a Focus on the Family chapel service several years earlier. Sandi Patti was the featured speaker. She only sang one song that morning which was unusual for this talented vocalist.

Just as I stepped into the tub, the soft background music began as she quoted Psalm 139, verses thirteen through sixteen—the exact verses I had marked in my Bible that spring. My ears perked up to hear the words she then sang to her daughter:

Before you had a name or opened up your eyes
Or anyone could recognize your face,
You were being formed so delicate in size
Secluded in God's safe and hidden place.
With your little tiny hands and little tiny feet
And little eyes that shimmer like a pearl,
He breathed in you a song and to make it all complete
He brought the masterpiece into the world.

You are a masterpiece,
A new creation He has formed
And you're as soft and fresh as a snowy winter morn.
And I'm so glad that God has given you to me
Little Lamb of God
You are a masterpiece.

And now you're growing up, your life's a miracle
Every time I look at you, I stand in awe
Because I see in you a reflection of me.
And you'll always be my little Lamb from God
And as your life goes on each day,
How I pray that you will see
Just how much your life has meant to me.
And I'm so proud of you
What else is there to say

Just be the masterpiece He created you to be.
You are a masterpiece,
A new creation He has formed
And you're as soft and fresh as a snowy winter morn.
And I'm so glad that God has given you to me
Little Lamb of God
You are a masterpiece. [1]

This was it! Without a doubt! The song for our baby—"Masterpiece." He had also re-confirmed the Psalm 139 verses. As I sat surrounded by bubbles in the tub that morning, with my stomach the biggest bubble of all, I thanked God for the precious life growing within me. What more did I need to know? God the Creator had told me that my baby was "fearfully and wonderfully made" and "a masterpiece."

Chapter Two

A Masterpiece?

November 10, 1991—due date. No arrival. November 11—the arrival on that day was my parents, Algie and Ruth Boone, as they drove in from McComb, Mississippi. I had spent my childhood years in that small southern town. Dad was from a family of eleven children, so our Boone family gatherings were frequent and large and spirited. We all went to church together. Twenty-five cousins made up a wonderful pool of playmates.

On daily walks my grandfather often visited six of his children's homes. And there were many Sunday dinners at my grandparents' house, followed by hours of play in the front yard. There was prayer at every family gathering. The inscription on Papa Boone's tombstone summed up the goal of the Boone clan: "Meet me in heaven." It was a secure setting. It took me years to realize how blessed I had been in childhood.

Dad was retired from years of sales—with Sears and a local automobile dealer. We teased him that he was the only honest car salesman we knew. Some thought Dad gruff at first, but anyone who knew him well saw his tender spirit. Tender toward his God, his wife, and his children.

Mother was a full-time homemaker. Her example had given me the desire to be at home with our children. It was always good to hear her soft southern drawl on our weekly phone calls. She was an organizer and a learner—teaching Sunday school and Bible studies. She had shared her thirst for books and learning with me.

Sterling greeted Grandpa and Grandma with warm hugs and slobbery kisses. I relaxed, knowing that he would be content in their care.

As they unloaded the car in the drive that Monday afternoon, Dad's first words were, "We're here. You can have the baby tonight."

Those words were repeated several times over the next week as we all eagerly waited.

By the following Monday, the only project left undone from my nesting list was planting pansies in the front flower beds. Pansies grow beautifully through the mild winters in the Dallas/Fort Worth area. They are typically planted in October and bloom through April when the heat returns.

I pictured the day Chuck and I would bring our new baby home from the hospital. As we turned off of busy Cummings Street into our quiet subdivision, we would first see the American flag waving atop the twenty-five foot flagpole in our front yard. Hanging just beneath the American flag would be the new baby's birthday flag. It was a tradition we had started when Sterling was born. On the day we brought him home from the hospital, there was a pale blue flag flying to welcome us home. "Happy Birthday, Sterling, February 2, 1990," the red, white and blue letters proclaimed. What a delightful surprise! Several weeks earlier Chuck had described his idea to Rhonda, a friend who was an excellent seamstress. She had designed and made the flag, adding the date and name as soon as he was born. We called her our family's Betsy Ross. We flew it that first week of his life, announcing his arrival to the neighborhood. On each birthday, it went up the flagpole for the day.

Rhonda had the new baby's flag as ready as possible. This one was royal blue, already bearing a red "Happy Birthday" and "November —, 1991." It only needed the date and name to be stitched in white. I imagined my first glimpse of it joyfully flying above the housetops as we brought the baby home from the hospital.

Rounding the corner on Willow Creek Drive we would see #3825, second house on the right, a two-story brick building—home to the

Watsons. We would pass the house, pull into the drive, stop at the front walkway, and see Sterling along with Grandpa and Grandma bounding out the front door to greet us. As we walked to the front door with the baby nestled in my arms, Sterling would show his new sibling the clusters of yellow pansies along the walkway.

"These are for you, baby. Sterling helped," he would explain.

Everything was in place for this scene except the flowers and the baby. The flowers were my project for that Monday. As I kissed Chuck good-bye at the back door that morning on his way to the office, I teasingly remarked, "I'll call you as soon as the pansies are planted. Then we can head for the hospital."

Dad, Mother, Sterling, and I headed to the redwood picnic table on the patio where seventy-two smiling yellow pansies awaited us. We made several trips to the front yard with the red wagon, loaded with flowers, spades, and fertilizer. Mother and Dad were still convinced that I could not and should not do this while nine plus months pregnant. But I had a need to do it as a part of my welcome to this little one.

"I'll just sit down on the sidewalk and stay down until I finish planting. You may need a crane to lift me when we finish, but I will be fine," I laughingly reassured them. "Maybe it will help bring on labor."

Dad dug the holes as I scooted along behind him, placing a plant in each hole. I did wish several times for one of those dollies that auto mechanics use to roll back and forth under cars. Mother trimmed the surrounding shrubs. Sterling played with the empty plant containers and dug extra holes. We stood back to survey our work with the bright pansies waving in the southern sunshine. My mother heart felt ready. The nest was complete.

"I think we'll be headed to the hospital tonight," I again assured everyone.

By Wednesday afternoon, even my patience had waned. As I lay on the table in Dr. Guthrie's office watching a sonogram with Chuck, my frustrations grew. It was time. It was past time. Was I going to be pregnant forever? The sonogram confirmed that the baby was ten days overdue and BIG. To my repeated questions of "How big?" the obstetrician's only response was, "Have you thought about a football player?"

"Everything looks fine, but the baby needs to come out," advised Dr. Guthrie. "I'm concerned about the need for a cesarean delivery if we wait any longer. In fact that may already be necessary. We'll induce labor first thing tomorrow. You need to be at the hospital by 5:30 in the morning."

It was a different feeling going to bed that night, *knowing* that I would be having a baby the next day. I thought this was the one date in your life that you couldn't plan, but I now knew my baby's birth date would be on Thursday, November 21, 1991. The only questions left—boy or girl (unanswered by our choice), and the time of day.

The next morning at 5:15, Chuck and I climbed the stairs to Sterling's bedroom. As I paused at the top to catch my breath, I was grateful that it was my last trip up those stairs "great with child." We held hands in the darkness by his crib as we prayed and kissed Sterling good-bye. It was an emotional moment for both of us, realizing that our family structure would never be the same again. This was the end of an era for him—no more "only child." Sterling lay peacefully sleeping, unaware of the upcoming transition.

As we tip-toed into the dining room at the bottom of the stairs, we found Grandma with her cup of coffee and Bible. She had gotten up to see us off with the loving anxiousness typical of a mother sending her daughter to the labor room. They've been there before, remember?

The three of us prayed together. After hugs and kisses, Chuck and I headed through the kitchen, out the back door, across the patio, and into the darkened garage. (Okay, maybe I waddled and he walked.) Suitcase in, people in, key in—and no response. The battery in the van was dead.

After a quick switch of luggage, people, and keys, we were on our way in my parents' car.

As we backed out of the drive, the thought crossed my mind that something was not right. I quickly dismissed it. God had already told me what I needed to know about this child—fearfully and wonderfully made, a masterpiece. On that cold November morning as we drove through the sleeping streets of Bedford, I knew that everything would be fine.

We arrived at Hurst-Euless-Bedford (HEB) Harris Methodist Hospital just eight minutes from home. I felt presumptuous presenting myself at the delivery desk, minus labor pains, with the announcement—"I'm here to have my baby."

We settled in at labor/delivery/recovery (LDR) suite number two. What a beautiful setting. The hardwood floors, elegant drapes, ash wooden furniture, classic paintings of females, soft floral sofa—this was a woman's room—the perfect decoration for a relaxing vacation. The sight of the hospital bed in the center of the room brought me back to reality.

Within minutes Chuck had the video camera perched on the tripod and ready for action. The cassette player was singing forth a gentle rendition of "Jesus Loves Me," and the framed words of Psalm 139:13-16 sat on the end table. We had printed the scripture on the computer and entitled it Baby Watson's Promise. It now boldly proclaimed to all who entered the room that this child was "fearfully and wonderfully made."

By 7:00 a.m. they had induced labor with the drug pitocin. Our nurse Jody was new at this hospital and still on probation, so all procedures had to be checked by someone else. But we had plenty of time—we would be there until this baby arrived! Jody was kind, although hesitant in her work, and had the same name as my childhood friend. I instantly liked her.

By 10:30 a.m. I welcomed the epidural (spinal anesthesia that deadens feeling from the waist down). I even napped through the lunch hour.

Shortly after that, Mother came by to visit for a few minutes. At 1:45 p.m. Chuck took a walk down the hallway and happened to meet Nancy, a favorite nurse who had been present at Sterling's delivery twenty-one months earlier. He brought her back to the LDR to say hello.

At 2:02 just as she was leaving the room, the baby's heart rate suddenly dropped from ninety beats per minute to sixty beats. Nancy went into action. She quickly turned me on my side while ordering Jody to call for the doctor "stat."

The nerves in my body started to come alive as the effects of the epidural waned. "It's time for more medicine in the epidural *now*," I reminded. "I'm feeling this more and more every minute."

"Sorry, but we can't give you anything with the baby's heart rate dropping. It's too risky since we're not sure what's going on." Nancy hustled about watching monitors and checking heartbeats.

Dr. Guthrie arrived at 2:12. They administered oxygen to me in hopes of helping the baby. Twelve minutes later, he used an emergency vacuum suction to get the baby out. It was 2:26 p.m.

Seconds later as Dr. Guthrie placed her on my stomach and we saw the first indications of breathing problems, my mind reeled. What was happening?

I kept telling myself that she just needed a little time to catch her breath. That it was nothing more than getting her system going after the cord being around her neck. "Is there a way to give her some oxygen?" I questioned. Surely that would fix everything.

At 2:30—four minutes into our daughter's life—Nancy returned to my bedside. "They're going to take her to the nursery and see how . . . and make sure everything is okay. She's still a little floppy. Her pulse is not good yet."

"Let Chuck see her again before she goes," I pleaded.

I could not see her although she was only a few feet away. Dr.

Guthrie was delivering the placenta and sewing me up without anesthesia. To say the least, I was aware of everything he was doing.

Chuck stood looking first at the baby, now bluer than before, and then at me, still shaking uncontrollably. "Do you want me to stay with you or go with the baby?" he asked.

"Go with her. Go with her," I begged.

Chuck and one of the nurses, with baby in arms, raced down the hallway to the nursery. There were frantic moments as they stood outside the door, unable to get in because of a new security system installed the previous day. The door now had a combination lock, and the nurse's memory blanked out as she stood holding this baby who continued to struggle for breath.

"Open the door. Get this door open," she barked to those inside.

Once inside the nursery, the baby was placed under an oxyhood to help with breathing. Chuck took this moment to sprint to the nearby maternity waiting room to tell Grandma Boone and my sister Rose Annette the news. "It's a girl. She's having trouble breathing. Pray!" They followed Chuck to the nursery and peeked through the mini blinds as the medical team feverishly worked over her.

Within minutes Pastor Jim and our friend Nancy arrived from the church office to join the line-up outside the nursery window. Months later they laughed at themselves as they described the scene—four adults crowded together at a two-foot window, stooping to see under the bottom edge of closed mini blinds, noses pressed against the window pane, and rear ends protruding into the hallway at a most interesting angle.

After a few minutes back in the nursery, Chuck realized that the baby was no better. At 2:40 he returned to the LDR suite to check on me. As he walked into the room, breathless yet trying to appear calm, he reported, "They're working. They're just trying to get her to breathe more regularly. She's going to be okay." At that point his voice broke. Tearfully he contin-

ued, "Dr. Terry (the hospital pediatrician) is there with the baby." His fear
of losing both of us was growing.

Nurse Nancy soothingly filled the silence. "Your church called again,
and they're praying."

We realized that God had sent Nancy across Chuck's path in the hallway moments before the birth. She was a ministering angel during those
frantic hours.

Chuck then continued, "They've got about four nurses, and there's
oxygen on the baby. The baby is screaming, so they're just getting her to
breathe more regularly."

Dr. Guthrie had left to get an update and returned with a new report.
It is best summarized by the hospital records: "Shortly after delivery, the
baby was noted to have marked respiratory difficulty, rapidly requiring
progression from an oxyhood to nasal CPAP (nasal tube-assisted breathing) to positive pressure ventilation (respirator). During her initial
work-up . . . chest x-ray revealed significant cardiomegaly (enlarged
heart) with granular appearance to both lung fields. The possibility of
congenital heart disease was raised." An emergency team was now en
route by helicopter to transport her to Cook Children's Medical Center
(CCMC) in Fort Worth for evaluation.

Chuck continued to rotate between the nursery and the LDR, keeping tabs on both of us. The transport team arrived at 3:35 and worked
with the nursery team for over an hour to stabilize her.

Nurse Nancy stayed at my bedside. During that hour, she gradually
prepared me for what I would see when they brought the baby to me on
her way to the ambulance. I had been given a sedative to stop the shaking
and was fighting to stay awake for this brief moment.

The LDR room was full—Chuck, Dad, Mother, Rose Annette, Nurse
Nancy—when four members of the CCMC emergency team wheeled in
the portable isolette. They opened down one side of the small glass box

to reveal my baby, sedated by morphine, with multiple tubes protruding from nose, mouth, and navel. Amid all the machinery and tubes, her nine-pound six-ounce body looked stuffed into the tiny bed typically used to transport two or three pound premature infants. The most I could do was raise up enough to touch her hand. Within seconds she was whisked away, and I was out. It was 4:44 p.m.

Grandma Boone rode with her in the ambulance. We originally thought they were transporting by helicopter when she agreed to go. This is a woman who hates to ride on big jets. Her agreeing to get on a helicopter was definitely a sacrifice of love!

By 7:00 that evening, Dr. Stephen Lai, pediatric cardiologist, telephoned from Fort Worth to give us the diagnosis. My hospital room was filled with family and friends as we listened breathlessly to Chuck's side of the conversation. It didn't sound good. Once again my entire body began to shake. Was *everything* out of control? Didn't I even have command over my own body?

When he hung up the phone, he turned to face a room of tearful people. For the first time I heard the words "Ebstein's Anomaly." This rare congenital heart defect is caused by a malformation of the tricuspid valve which pumps the blood from the heart's upper right chamber (atrium) to the lower right chamber. Because the valve was not pumping the blood forward through the heart, her right atrium had filled with blood sloshing backward through the valve opening. That chamber was now enlarged six to seven times its original size, filling her chest cavity and pressing on her lungs. Dr. Lai's written report concluded: "Newborn girl . . . with huge tricuspid valve insufficiency. Greatly enlarged right atrium accounts for the child's cardiomegaly (enlarged heart) on x-ray."

Medical books summarize Ebstein's Anomaly in this way:

"Treatment. Treatment of this condition in the newborn

is based on two premises: (1) many infants improve markedly over the first weeks of life, presumably as the pulmonary vascular resistance drops, and (2) surgical approaches to treating the critically ill newborn have thus far been almost uniformly unsuccessful.

"Prognosis. The prognosis is worse for patients presenting in the newborn period. In an international collaborative study, 29 of 35 infants died."[2]

That's a seventeen percent survival rate for newborns. Everyone joined hands, encircling my bed, and we prayed. In my hands I clutched a Polaroid snapshot of the baby, taken by a nurse moments before she had been transferred. It was my only tangible connection to her. I longed to hold her, to comfort her, to let her hear my familiar voice, to make everything right for her. I felt robbed of those first bonding moments, and now she was fighting for life twenty-five miles away. My biggest concern was that she be peaceful. I had to know that she wasn't frightened.

After a powerful prayer time, Chuck, Grandpa Boone, and a friend Mark headed to the baby and Grandma in Fort Worth. I sent several cassette tapes to play by her bedside—one of soft Christian lullabies and another of her song "You Are A Masterpiece."

———————— ⟫⟫⟩ ————————

Baby Watson had her first heart-to-heart talk with her Daddy that night. He checked out every detail to make sure that she was as comfortable as possible. Then he remained by her bedside until 1:30 a.m.

When Chuck returned to my room at 2:00 a.m., I was weary yet bursting with questions. "Is she peaceful? Are you sure she's not frightened? Is she any better? Has anything changed?"

Yes, she was peaceful. No, nothing had changed. I moved to my next pressing concern. "I'm tired of everyone referring to her as Baby Watson. It sounds so impersonal. We've got to name her. I know we wanted to hold her in our arms when we named her, but we can't wait for that. I'm just disappointed that we can't even look at her while we choose her name," I confided. Once again I felt robbed.

My dear husband, a man of detail even in the midst of crisis, pulled a video tape from underneath his jacket. "I filmed her while I was down there so that you could see her in her surroundings. I thought this would be helpful in naming her."

Minutes later a nurse arrived in the room pushing a cart loaded with a VCR and television. I pulled out the list of names with their meanings that we had compiled over the past months. As Chuck turned on the video, the list of names fluttered to my lap forgotten as I froze, mesmerized by the images on the screen.

Her bed looked like an open glass box about two feet long. The clear sides were ten inches high. Two wallet-sized photos were taped to the inner side of the bed—our wedding photo and Sterling's eighteen-month picture. Machines surrounded the bed, which sat on a stand with wheels, bringing the bed height to Chuck's waist. Tubes snaked their way onto the bed from every direction. As I followed those tubes, they all converged on my daughter's body.

At the top of the bed, three respirator tubes arched upward over her head and joined just above her eyes to form a single large tube that went into her mouth. Tape covered the lower portion of her face from ear to ear, crossing above her upper lip, and holding the tube in place. Another smaller tube went from her nose to a baby bottle lying on the bed. A bottle! One normal thing! But no, this one contained the acid and air being drained from her stomach. Three round patches on her chest were each connected to wires leading to a heart monitor. I tracked another tube from her navel to a pole containing a pouch of IV fluid—her first meal. Something similar to a tiny band-aid was wrapped around one of her toes. A red light flashed from the "band-aid," and its wire led to yet another machine that measured the amount of oxygen she was getting in her system. Overhead another machine monitored the temperature of the bed. I heard the steady soft beep of each heartbeat registered by the monitor. In the background people were talking and other monitors beeped.

My eyes filtered their way through the machines, tubes, and noises to find my daughter. She lay on her back, clothed only with tape and tubes. Her puffy body (due to fluid accumulation) looked like a war zone. Curly dark hair covered her head and faded into a blue forehead. Her swollen eyelids were closed. The outstretched arms ended in clenched fists which were also blue. The insertion sight for the tube going into her navel looked nasty. It was easy to see the struggle within as I watched her chest heave up and down with each breath. Repeatedly, her body trembled.

At her right side stood Grandpa, clothed in a white gown and mask. He and Chuck prayed for her softly. Grandpa then operated the camera while Chuck moved to her side. It was a precious scene. He took the fingers of her right hand and wrapped them around his giant index finger. With his other hand he gently stroked the front of her hand as he softly sang "Jesus Loves Me." Her eyes opened briefly. With a puzzled look, those huge blue eyes sought for the source of that familiar voice, and then closed again.

"Angel, you are so beautiful." Chuck's voice comforted her. "Your hands . . . your face . . . your legs . . . your feet. You kept putting those feet in Mommy's chest. You are a special girl. Daddy loves you. Mommy loves you. Sterling, your big brother, loves you. You are so pretty . . . I have another song to play for you. Mommy sent it down here. It's *your* song."

As the music began, Sandi Patti spoke the now familiar words of Psalm 139:13-16:

You made my whole being;
You formed me in my mother's body.
You saw my bones being formed
as I took shape in my mother's body.
When I was put together there,
You saw my body as it was formed.
I praise You
because You made me
in an amazing and wonderful way.

She then sang—

Before you had a name or opened up your eyes
Or anyone could recognize your face,
You were being formed so delicate in size
Secluded in God's safe and hidden place.
With your little tiny hands and little tiny feet
And little eyes that shimmer like a pearl,
He breathed in you a song and to make it all complete
He brought the masterpiece into the world.

You are a masterpiece,
A new creation He has formed
And you're as soft and fresh as a snowy winter morn.
And I'm so glad that God has given you to me
Little Lamb of God
You are a masterpiece. [1]

The music continued on with the second verse, but I didn't hear. To watch her suffer was difficult enough. But hearing those words of scripture, and that song, was like rubbing salt into an open wound. I felt like the brunt of a cruel inhumane joke. Blocking out the music, I looked only at my precious baby. My mothers heart ached, watching her fight for life with me miles away and unable to go to her.

What my eyes saw on the video, and what my ears heard in the song and scripture, did not match. Talk about a contradiction! Who was I to think that I would have a healthy baby? Who said it would be different this time? This made Sterling's illness look easy!

When the video ended, I shoved my questions into a dark inner corner. The conflict was too much for me. Those questions would have to come later. At that moment, the one thing I could do for my daughter was to give her a name.

Chuck and I had not had a chance to discuss names from our list since her birth, but we quickly discovered that the same name had been on each of our minds throughout the afternoon—Heidi Joy. Our research showed that "Heidi" means "of noble character." That's a good meaning, but we had wanted something with a little more power behind it for the battle that might be ahead. But "Heidi" felt right. We had been fairly certain of a girl's middle name for months. "Heidi Joy." We both felt strongly that this was the name for this child.

At that moment, it was the *only* thing in my life that I knew was right!

Chapter Three

It Wasn't Supposed To Be This Way

Day three of Heidi's life. On that Saturday morning, I awakened at HEB Hospital in Bedford, relieved that I would be released and could finally go to my baby in Fort Worth. Rose Annette had spent the night on the floor in my tiny room to give Chuck a night's rest.

It was always good to be with my sister, but especially now. My memories with her went back to her own birth when I was four years old. I had helped name her. My parents had chosen the name Rose after my maternal grandmother. They allowed six-year-old Danny and me to select her middle name. Remember the Mickey Mouse Club? She was named after our favorite mouseketeer—Annette Funicello.

We sisters were as opposite as day and night. She's shorter, I'm taller. She's blonde (an authentic one!), I'm brunette. As a child she was the outgoing life of the party, while I was a shy bookworm.

On one family vacation, we had stopped to get gasoline and couldn't find Rose Annette when we were ready to leave. We finally discovered her visiting with the people in the car behind us. After a reminder from Daddy and Mother about strangers, she replied, "Oh, they're not strangers. They live in Louisiana. The woman is a school teacher, and they are on their way to Michigan. They're going camping with their family. They were very nice. I told them all about our family." Like Dad, she never met a stranger.

In adult life, Rose Annette and I had switched roles somewhere along the way. She was now the quieter one, and I the more outgoing. However, I had not reached the point of exchanging family histories at gasoline pumps!

We were different and yet very close in spirit. Growing up, the four year age difference had been wide. In our adult years, it blurred to nothing. For a year we shared an apartment together as single women in Kansas City. I was blessed with good female roommates during my single years, but she was my favorite. We became very close during that time. There was little money, but an abundance of friends and fun.

She always made sure people knew she was younger, although she had entered some seasons ahead of me, most notably marriage and children. It was in Kansas City that I had introduced her to my best buddy Bryan. I had told her they would be perfect for each other. They were equally unimpressed upon meeting and married a year and a half later! Now she and Bryan lived eight minutes away with eight-year-old Jeremy and six-year-old Jessica.

The "sister talk" interspersed throughout the night as we awakened had been a soothing balm. It helped prepare me for the day ahead.

It was a sunny day. Other mothers were also leaving the hospital. But they were going home *with* their babies. They had been cuddling newborns in their arms for the past two days. I had been clutching a Polaroid photograph of Heidi as I hourly received medical reports of her worsening condition. They had been feeding their babies. Last night I had turned up the volume of my music so I couldn't hear the healthy cries of newborns feeding in the neighboring rooms. I took no walks down the hall to the nursery window. I had been telephoning the NICU (Neonatal Intensive Care Unit) nurses miles away to ask about Heidi.

This wasn't the way it was supposed to be! Was this really happening? Or was it a terrible nightmare that I would awaken from at any moment? Pregnant women go to the hospital, have healthy babies, and bring those babies home triumphantly. Yet I was going home to an empty cradle at the foot of our bed. But my baby was alive. I had to stay focused on that point.

As I slowly dressed that morning, I looked forward to one thing—seeing Heidi. Chuck, Dad, Rose Annette, and I were stepping over each other in our efforts to get us packed and out of there. Mother was at home caring for Sterling.

I managed to shower and dress before my energy waned. Leaning against the dresser, I tried to summon the energy to do make-up and hair. The phone rang. It was Cook's Hospital telling us to come right away. Heidi was in trouble. If we wanted to see her, we needed to come immediately. Chuck summoned the nurse and signed dismissal papers. Rose Annette stayed behind to pack my bags. Dad stayed to jump start the van which once again refused to start. This time it was in the hospital parking lot.

A nurse arrived with a wheelchair, and Chuck and I started the long trip to the car. Long not in distance, but in emotions. As we turned the corner from the short hallway onto the long main corridor of the maternity unit, I saw the other rooms. Then I understood. They had told us the tiny corner room was the only thing available, although the hospital hadn't appeared to be full. But I had been mercifully placed at the end of the unit down a side hallway to be away from the sights and sounds of babies as much as possible.

As we passed, some doors were open revealing glowing new mothers. Many doors had wreaths decked with bears and streamers joyously announcing "It's a boy" or "It's a girl." I was reminded again of the painful difference between my experience of the past two days and that of the other mothers.

As the nurse pushed the wheelchair, Chuck walked slowly at my side hurting in two different ways—feeling his own pain as a father, and feeling helpless as he watched me hurt. Wheeling down the hall, my overwhelming thought was, *God, please don't let me see another baby. Don't make me watch another lady leave here with a newborn nestled in her arms.*

We were halfway down the hall when Chuck abruptly commanded the nurse—"Turn right here. We're going this way."

The nurse hesitated, confused as to why we wouldn't take the most direct route, but followed his authoritative lead. I knew. He was doing everything possible to get us out of there without intercepting another mother and child.

As we rounded the final corner, the outside door was in sight. Ahead and to my left, I saw the back of a woman seated in a wheelchair. *Please, God, don't let there be a baby on her lap!* I pleaded inwardly. As we wheeled closer, I focused my eyes on the door, refusing to look her way. Her husband had pulled the car up to the door and was entering through the revolving door. Our wheelchairs were beside each other before I got the courage to glance her way. It was empty—there was no baby on her lap. Relief. *Thank you, God!* Then came the guilt. Oh no, I hoped she hadn't gone through what we were going through—or worse, lost her baby.

Dad pulled his car to the covered drive and stood waiting with the car door open. The cold November wind stung my cheeks as I shuffled out. Chuck placed the donut cushion (the "inner tube" pillow that new mothers sit on after delivery because of stitches) on the seat and gingerly helped me in. Silently the two of us started our first of many drives to Fort Worth. At that moment, all I wanted was for Heidi to live until we could get to her.

Although Saturday traffic was lighter, the drive seemed to take hours. Didn't people understand? Our baby was dying. Couldn't they at least move over?

Thirty minutes later, we were finally there. Cook Children's Medical Center. The setting reminded me of Disney's Magic Kingdom Castle. Shrubs lining the front drive were shaped like playful bears and dancing rabbits. Several fountains bubbled their waters into a large circular pool.

Just behind the pool under the covered drive, a brown van carried its cargo of balloons, stuffed animals, and a newly released child. The six-story white building glistened. Bright blue window frames and triangular cones atop each section of the building accented its shining white exterior.

Although I had protested that I did not need one, we drove around to the back of the hospital and entered through the emergency room where we could get a wheelchair. I tried to picture Heidi's arrival here two days earlier, probably through these same doors.

Through the corridors to the front of the hospital and up the elevator to the second floor—would we ever get there? A small, quiet chapel was near the elevator. It would become a haven for me in the days ahead. As we rounded the corner to the NICU waiting room, the quiet of the chapel seemed miles away. This looked like an overgrown living room. Five blue sofas faced each other, holding several family groups. One set of dazed young parents sat with their parents. Another couple huddled together, talking quietly. Two couples were laughing as they enjoyed lunch. Coffee tables held the remains of Burger King® lunches and newspapers. A young man sat talking on the telephone as his wife hovered by his side.

The father of the quiet couple greeted Chuck and asked about Heidi. "Not good," was his only reply. He shared my anxiousness to get to her. We stopped on the far side of the room near two large swinging doors. Chuck picked up a wall telephone and said, "This is Chuck and Vickie Watson. We're here to see Heidi. Can we come in?"

He seemed at home after only two days. I felt as if I had been jettisoned to another planet. We have to ask permission to see our daughter? My instincts told me to sprint back to the space shuttle and blast off for Earth—to return to my familiar world. But my baby was somewhere on this planet. So I was stuck here. I couldn't leave without her.

By the time we started through the maze of corridors hidden behind the double doors, I was totally disoriented. Me, the one who can find anyplace with a map, and retrace my steps without the map. Leaving the wheelchair in the waiting room, I followed Chuck like a robot in slow motion. All I could think about in my numbness was that behind one of these doors was my baby. I just wanted to find her and get us all out of there.

After several turns, he opened a heavy door and waited for me to enter. It was a large brightly lit room. Here was the command post of this strange planet—the NICU, Side A, Critical Care. The room was divided into four rows, with each aisle containing six isolettes. Machinery lined the shelves above each bed. Each row ended at a window-lined wall.

The sounds seemed louder than on the video. The beeping of the monitors, the blaring alarms, the whooshing of respirators as they breathed for these infants. Chuck had told me there were twelve babies in the unit. And yet the silence slapped at me. How can you have twelve infants in a room and yet hear no human sounds—no wails, no fussies, no burps? Babies on respirators make no sounds. They may be screaming, but you won't know it unless you look at their faces. I vowed at that moment to never complain again about the sound of a baby crying.

This was an eerie world of whooshing machinery and beeping monitors. The sounds reminded me of a muted boiler room. At the opposite end of the room, I saw another entrance with an office area just inside the door. Three nurses chatted at the desk while several others tended to infants.

Chuck directed me to the row of deep sinks. It was time for Scrubbing 101. Rings and watches off. Turn on water with lever beside your knee. Hands and lower arms washed for three minutes with antibacterial cleanser. Rinse under hot water. Turn off water with knee. Don't touch faucets. Put on hospital gown from the shelf behind you. No food or drinks allowed. Did I understand? I didn't even know how to get back to the car! My mind was not computing. Except for one thought. *Where is my baby?* I was blindly going through whatever motions it took to get to Heidi.

As Chuck led me down the first aisle I started a "bed search." *No, not in the first one. Only a cluster of machines surrounding that bed.* Then I froze momentarily. Yes, there *was* a baby in that bed. At the center of those wires laid an infant no bigger than the palm of my hand. He weighed one pound fifteen ounces. I was not ready for this. *Okay, stare straight ahead until Chuck shows you Heidi's bed,* I commanded inwardly as my weak knees carried me further into the room.

Past another bed, turn to the left, then to the right, down aisle number two. We stopped at the last bed next to the window. There she was, face turned toward the window. There was no medical team hovering over her. That was a good sign. I quickly moved around the bed to see her face.

"Heidi," I whispered, "it's Mommy." Frightened eyes looked up at me as I inserted my little finger into her clenched fist.

"She's scared. You told me she was peaceful. And she's not," I sobbed. "She is so afraid. Don't you see it?" I lashed out at Chuck as if it were his fault. He was the only one present to blame.

"Honey, she has been peaceful when I've been here. You know I would have told you. You'll see it in her eyes later. I promise."

Heidi's nurse came over to introduce herself and update us. She explained that Heidi's oxygen levels had worsened throughout the morning. That's the amount of oxygen breathed in that gets to our body for use. Our oxygen saturation level is 100%. The written medical report stated, "Oxygen sats mostly in 60's, dipping into 50's at times . . . Infant remains pale, with duskiness on feet, hands, lips." She was getting barely more than half the oxygen she needed. Yet the numbers didn't even register with me. Tears continued to roll down my cheeks as I stared at Heidi.

I hadn't even seen the nurse's face.

"Do you have any questions?" she asked.

I only had one—"Why is that card with the number seven hanging above her bed?" It must have seemed totally irrelevant to her. My daughter was dying, and I was asking about numbers taped on the shelves. I had noticed it on the video Thursday night when we named Heidi.

"She is in bed number seven within the unit," she explained. That was what I was hoping to hear. Seven is God's perfect number. Couldn't that at least count for something? Could that be a sign that God was working here? I was grasping for anything.

The nurse started to leave, then turned back toward us. "Mr. and Mrs. Watson, I want to help you put this in perspective. Heidi looks the healthiest of any baby in here. She dwarfs the others with her nine - pound six-ounce, fluid-filled body. Don't let that fool you. She is the sickest baby we have." Although delivered gently, the words stung. They snapped me out of the fog.

"Heidi, this is Mommy. Daddy and I are here with you, and everything's going to be okay. It's not always going to be this hard. Just hang in there. Life will get easier. We are fighting with you. You don't need to be afraid. We're going to make it together."

I wasn't sure that what I said was true—the part about life getting easier. Hopefully Heidi didn't sense that. If either of us could have read the cardiologist's report written a few hours earlier, we would have been even more unsure. "Prognosis remains in doubt at this time."

Chuck was called to the hospital business office to complete more paperwork. His ability to shift gears astounded me. One minute he could be singing to Heidi, then discussing her case with the nurse, then praying for her, then meeting the doctor on call that weekend, then tearfully encouraging Heidi and telling her of his love.

I was stuck in one gear—numb, with one question. *How can I get my baby out of here?* For several hours, I perched on the stool by her side, our fingers glued together.

It must have been traumatic to go from the cozy security of the womb to lying spread-eagled on her back in a brightly lit room. If only I could snuggle her and rock her in my arms. But the tubes, IVs, and wires stood between her body and my embrace. Fingers and kisses were our limit.

Then I remembered something Rose Annette had told me in the wee hours of that morning. She and Bryan had spent that Friday evening with Heidi before coming to my hospital. Rose Annette had experienced the same desire to hold Heidi and comfort her. So they placed their arms along each side of her from head to foot, nestling each side of her head within their hands. And Heidi got her first hug from Uncle Bryan and Auntie Rose.

When Chuck returned from the office, we tried it. He once again assured me, "Vickie, we're going to do what works for Heidi. The hugs and care may be different for awhile, but we're going to take care of her. We'll know how to do it." His confidence, even in the midst of this new world, bolstered my weary emotions.

By mid-afternoon, Chuck knew it was time for us to go. "Right now you've got to get some rest, or you won't be able to help Heidi."

He was right. But would I see her again? Or would they call us once again to rush to her side? Would we get there soon enough if that happened? It was so hard to leave.

The three of us prayed together. Just before leaving, I whispered, "Heidi, we'll be back tomorrow. Grandma Watson is flying here from Ohio right now. She and Grandma Boone will spend the night with you tonight. And Jesus is always with you. You don't have to be afraid. We love you. Good night."

With stitches burning after several hours of sitting, and heart aching at leaving her again, I headed home.

Home. It sounded so good. But that brought pain also. Heidi's birthday flag. I saw it above the rooftops before we turned the corner. How could it flap in the breeze? It should have been motionless at least for this moment. Yellow pansies in the front yard. They mockingly danced as we walked past them into the house. Who was I to think that I would have a healthy baby? How presumptuous of me!

In our bedroom, the white Williamsburg cradle sat motionless at the foot of our bed. It was empty, except for the fluffy stuffed lamb that Sterling had placed in one corner and the ripple-stitch baby afghan folded neatly across the bottom. Grandma Boone had crocheted the pale pink, blue, green, and yellow yarns into a beautiful heirloom in preparation for her seventh grandchild. The cradle was going to be empty for awhile. Maybe forever? *Please God, no!*

I stumbled to our bed and crawled in, pausing only long enough to kick off my shoes. Pulling the down comforter over my head, I was hoping to shut out everything, including my thoughts. I was back on familiar turf, but that only made the truth clearer. Today we had come home from the hospital without our baby. The doctors told us that she probably would not live. And her condition was worsening by the day. **God, it wasn't supposed to be this way!**

Chapter Four

THE BATTLE PLAN

It was twenty-one-month-old Sterling who brought me out from under the covers hours later. Having just awakened from his nap, he came toddling to my bedside with a quiet, "Ma-ma-ma." He seemed to have grown up in the three days since I had seen him. It's amazing how a newborn will make your other child look older. It felt good to hug and kiss and giggle together.

Chuck pulled the large gift-wrapped box out of my closet. "This is from baby Heidi to you, Sterling," he explained. "We're all excited that you are a big brother now."

We spent the next half hour playing airplanes with his new Fisher-Price airport set. It was a toss-up as to which Sterling enjoyed more—the airplane or the big box.

Late that evening, the household gathered for dinner. Grandma Watson had arrived in the afternoon. It was still strange seeing her without Grandpa who had died a year and a half earlier. There were six of us around the oak kitchen table—Grandpa and Grandma Boone, Grandma Watson, Chuck, Sterling, and me. Delicious food had been provided by a church family. Within minutes of blessing the meal, it was apparent to all that Chuck was gearing up for action. Always the man with a plan. Never one to waste time beating around the bush. My first bite was still in my mouth when he started:

"We need to lay out a plan for Heidi's hospital stay. She needs some of us with her around the clock. She needs our emotional support and our prayers continually by her side. I'm thinking that three eight-hour shifts per day would work best. The two grandmas could share the night shift at the hospital from 11:00 p.m. to 7:00 a.m.; Grandpa Boone and a daily substitute grandpa in place of my dad would take the daytime hours from 7:00 a.m. to 3:00 p.m.; and Vickie and I would be there from 3:00 p.m. to 11:00 p.m. That would also give Vickie some daytime hours with Sterling to keep his life as normal as possible."

I knew his thinking without hearing it voiced. He realized that neither of us was ready to handle the hospital without each other. Especially me without him right then. We desperately needed each other.

He continued: "So one shift will be with Heidi at the hospital, one shift with Sterling at home, and one shift sleeping. When you're with Heidi, if you don't know what to do after talking to her, then read the Bible to her or play the worship tapes. Anytime you leave her side, be sure there is Christian music playing.

"Dad, I've lined up men for several days next week to be at the hospital with you. I'm expecting calls from others this evening.

"I had already requested vacation time for next week because of Thanksgiving, so I won't have to worry about my work schedule until the first of December. Hopefully Heidi will be home by then.

"I talked to Pastor Jim this afternoon by phone. Tomorrow morning they'll show some of our video footage of Heidi during the church service. Many already know and have been praying. But there will be a church-wide time of prayer on her behalf tomorrow. Church families are bringing meals each evening, and daily volunteers will answer our phone, giving reports on Heidi's condition and keeping the prayer chain updated. That should help us get more rest when we are here. They have offered to provide anything else we need.

"So what do you think of the plan?"

I sat in stunned silence. God had clearly given Chuck the working details for the battle ahead. How grateful I was for a husband gifted with administrative abilities and wisdom from God. This was a starting point to get us through the days ahead. It sounded great.

———— ⬛➤ ————

My part in the battle plan did not become clear until the following Monday. It had been a difficult weekend with Heidi's condition continuing to worsen. There had been no improvement in any area since her birth.

There is a small ductus between the two upper chambers of the heart which is open during the prenatal period of life. At birth or within the first week of life, this ductus naturally closes. Once it closes, it cannot be reopened. This open ductus had been helping pump some of the blood out of Heidi's vastly enlarged right atrium (upper heart chamber).

On Sunday it became apparent that the ductus was starting to close. Her heart could not yet function with that ductus closed. The right ventricle (lower heart chamber) could not compensate.

An emergency heart medication "prostaglandin" was started that afternoon to keep the ductus open. The doctors had been saving it as a last resort. Because of bad side effects, it is used only in emergency situations. I did not know until later that one of those effects is making you feel as if tiny bugs are crawling all over your body. That explained why she required so much more morphine during those days.

The plan was to wean her off the respirator and then stop the prostaglandin. She could not be on this medication for an extended time. The prostaglandin kept her ductus open and bought us a little more time for her to hopefully improve and come off the respirator. Dr. Smith, the neonatologist, summarized the situation in his written report: "Prognosis remains guarded."

I had expected and hoped for more from Sunday. Many church

bodies were physically together and praying for Heidi that day. Late that Sunday night we had watched the video of our own church's morning service. It was powerful!

I caught snatches of Pastor Jim's explanation of the situation as I tried to make my tired mind concentrate on the video:

> I bring you a rather urgent prayer request . . . a precious little girl, Heidi Joy . . . difficulty regards a deformed heart . . . is quite literally clinging to life this day . . . many of you have been there and prayed with them . . . also stiffening of the lungs and they're not functioning as they're supposed to . . . tremendous blood build up . . . she's in extremely critical condition . . . on numerous machines . . . a tremendously difficult time for Chuck and Vickie . . . it's not an overstatement to say that medical science cannot bring what we need right now . . . it's a matter of day by day staying alive . . . genuinely a life and death situation . . . the health problems with Sterling have been extensive . . . net result is a very tired family and very sleep-deprived family . . . When this baby was born with this complication, it was just almost more than two humans can bear. It really is more. We need to step in as a church and lift this family and particularly this little baby girl, Heidi Joy, in prayer . . . this is going to be an unusual day . . . we're going to focus on this little girl for the next few moments . . . we do have a brief video tape to give you a feel for what she looks like there in the hospital . . . we have much to do in this time of prayer . . . putting a stop to the work of the enemy . . . coming against fear in a moment like this

. . . coming against even doubt.

My eyes roamed the platform. Where was the choir? There were only nine robed choir members sprinkled across the risers. Then I realized— they were on their knees weeping, ready to cry out to God in prayer for our daughter!

I saw Jeff, one of the few choir members standing, and my heart ached for him. I wanted to help him escape from that service. Only eleven months earlier, his fiancée had been in an auto accident while on her way to pick out her wedding dress. This vibrant young woman in her early twenties lay in a coma for a month. As a church body we prayed. We stood. We battled. And she died. It had been a jolt to the faith of all of us.

And six months later, a member of the worship team, another woman in her early twenties, had committed suicide. That had caused much painful soul-searching in us as a body of believers. Where had we missed it in ministering to her? I certainly understood why the pastor was talking about battling doubt. We as a congregation needed to win one. And this time, it was my daughter. Our track record on big-time healing was not encouraging. How would this one end?

Pastor Jim's words echoed my thoughts:

> As you see the video I don't want you to be intimi-
> dated by all the hospital equipment . . . I want you to see
> Jesus standing there in the midst, touching her right
> now . . . **We really need to be with the Lord and see a
> victory now!**

Tearfully the pastor began to pray:

We are a people with a heavy heart. Our confidence is in You. We bring You what appears to be an insurmountable need from our standpoint. There is only One we can run to in this moment. We believe we would come to You even if there were other places to go. But there is no other place to go and we know that. We come to You—the only One who is capable of bringing the correction to this precious little heart that would cause it to work in the way in which You originally intended and designed it . . . We ask for your completion of this as we stand together as a church against every attack of the evil one in this moment. Driving back every way in which the enemy could make intrusion into this precious little one. Calling upon an angelic force to overshadow her right now even this moment in the hospital room.

As he paused in his prayer I recognized Henry's voice and my eyes spotted his silver hair and goatee as he knelt on the platform. This seventy-seven-year-old prophet had walked with God through many experiences, including a missionary term in Africa and the loss of a child. Still very much alive and kicking, Henry was always ready to share something new that he had recently learned. He raised his left arm with conviction as he spoke the words of the Lord:

Call upon Me in the day of trouble and I will hear thee and thou shalt glorify Me. God is able to do exceeding abundantly above all that we ask or think according to the power that worketh in us. Oh Lord, I ask you to work the power that works in us—that works in me. Because You can do anything. You are the great physician!

There was a steady stream of people coming forward to share God's Word. Although I couldn't see her on the video, I quickly recognized my dear friend Adrienne's voice:

> Psalm 147:12 says, "Praise the Lord, O Jerusalem! Praise your God, O Zion! For He has strengthened the bars of your gates." The gates are the valves. "He has blessed your children within you. He makes peace in your borders; He satisfies you with the finest of the wheat. He sends forth His command to the earth; His word runs very swiftly." And Isaiah 43:18 and 19 read, "Do not call to mind the former things, or ponder things of the past. Behold, I will do something new, now it will spring forth; will you not be aware of it? I will even make a roadway in the wilderness, rivers in the desert. The beasts of the field will glorify Me; the jackals and the ostriches; because I have given waters in the wilderness and rivers in the desert, to give drink to My chosen people. The people whom I formed for Myself will declare My praise." (Psalm 147:12-14; Isaiah 43:18-21, NASB)

Next was Laura, a busy young mother of three toddlers:

> The week before Heidi was born, I was reading this and felt I needed to call Vickie and share it with her. It's from Isaiah 49: "The Lord called me from the womb;

from the body of my mother He named me. And He has
made my mouth like a sharp sword; in the shadow of
His hand He has concealed me, and He has also made
me a select arrow; He has hidden me in His quiver. And
He said to me, 'You are My Servant, Israel, in whom I
will show My glory.'" (Isaiah 49:1b-3, NASB)

Doug, one of the care shepherds and a man always ready to see a miracle, read of a young boy's healing from Matthew 17:14:

"When they came to the crowd, a man approached
Jesus and knelt before Him. 'Lord, have mercy on my
son,' he said. 'He is an epileptic and is suffering greatly.
He often falls into the fire or into the water. I brought
him to Your disciples but they could not heal him.' 'Oh
unbelieving and perverse generation,' Jesus replied. '. . .
How long shall I put up with you? Bring the boy here to
me.' Jesus rebuked the demon, and it came out of the
boy, and he was healed from that moment. Then the disciples came to Jesus in private and asked, 'Why couldn't
we drive it out?' He replied, 'Because you have so little
faith. I tell you the truth, if you have faith as small as a
mustard seed, you can say to this mountain, "Move from
here to there" and it will move. Nothing will be impossible for you.'" (Matthew 17:14-21, NIV)

Father God, in the name of Jesus we get in agreement with Your Word. For Your Word does not return
unto you void, but it accomplishes the purposes where-
in you sent it. And we bring little Heidi Joy to you,
Jesus. And we say to You, "Our hope is in You. Our life

is in You. We put our trust in You. We bring her unto You." Father, Your Word says that they brought many unto Jesus and He healed them all. And right now as we see that little picture of Heidi Joy on the wall, we bring her and put her into Your hands. We get in agreement with Your Word. And it says because we've had so little faith, nothing was done. But when you speak to this mountain, the mountain of difficulty, the mountain of difficulty in her heart, nothing will be impossible to you. So we speak to that heart and we say, "Be whole in the name of Jesus." We say, "Valve form in the name of Jesus." We say, "Tissue grow. Valve form. All three layers of valve come forth now in the name of Jesus." We speak the Word into that heart. We say, "Be whole in the name of Jesus. Be complete in the name of Jesus." For the glory and the power of Your name. We give You praise, oh God. We say to Heidi Joy, "Be healed in Jesus' name." Hallelujah! Hallelujah!

As the camera panned to the right, there was a cluster of people around Pastor Travis waiting to speak into the microphone which he held. I was shocked to see Bob standing there. His son and daughter-in-law were close friends of ours. Bob was an outgoing man, tall and robust with a thick head of white hair. He was very intent on succeeding in business. Although outgoing one-on-one, I had never heard him speak in a public church service. I would not have believed the words were from Bob had I not heard them with my own ears:

   . . . I want to just give a word of testimony. You know there is a time in one's life when you set your

goals. You want to succeed and be successful. But I got
my eyes too much on being successful. I got my eyes on
too much of business. And I became lukewarm. But I
want to tell you all something. There are needs in this
church. There are men here today that, believe me, Jesus
is just waiting for you. He's right there. And all you have
to do is just come to Him with a broken and contrite
heart and say, "Jesus, I'm sorry. I've gotten my priorities
out of line."

His shoulders shook as he wept in brokenness before continuing:

> I want to praise Him. The other night . . . I rededi-
> cated my life to Jesus. I've never had such peace because,
> folks, you cannot buy the peace. Money is not the
> answer. Your goals in life and the materials are not the
> answer. **Jesus Christ is the answer.** The peace inside of
> you is worth everything. And if you've got that, you can
> stand on the Word. You can come against these things.
> You can speak to those mountains and they have to be
> removed because Jesus promised us that.

The congregation broke into applause. In the background I heard
several male voices encouraging him with "Right on!" Bob continued:

> It's not what we can do as individuals. But I want to
> tell you something. If you're lined up with the Word, if
> you're lined up with Jesus, there isn't anything that can
> come against us. Nothing can stop us as far as spiritual
> matters are concerned. And Satan can't either, man,

because we have strength over him and power over him through the precious blood of Jesus Christ. I love him dearly this morning. Praise His Name!

What a powerful exhortation. Pastor Jim directed the congregation in how to apply it:

> We've been challenged . . . to make sure we're in alignment with the will of God . . . We've heard the Word of the Lord that was spoken through Bob. And His Word was a strong one . . . that Jesus Christ is number one in our lives. You show me a congregation that <u>lives</u> that way, orders lives that way, and we <u>will</u> be able to pray prayers of faith that produce results. But show me a congregation that is half-hearted and has one foot stuck in the world, and it will be a church that prays prayers that do not have much effect.
>
> So there's a key to the promises of God and Bob has hit the nail right on the head. That we're a people who walk in conformity. When he spoke that word just now, that was designed for some of you . . . If you are willing to receive that as a Word from the Lord and bring correction into your own life, the Spirit of God will bring a re-prioritizing . . . Just raise your hand wherever you are . . . We can't pray an effective prayer as a church and get babies in hospitals healed, unless we're walking with our total selves thrown in at the altar of Christ. We don't keep a foot in the world and pray effective prayers. Impure churches don't pray very powerfully. Okay, numbers of you have raised your hands.

Father, you see these hands that have been raised. We come in a spirit of repentance and we ask for renewing. We ask for a cleansing of our own priorities, our lifestyles, our thoughts, our habit patterns. We ask for a purging and a purifying of each and every sin. We ask every sin to be cast out before we're going to ask for babies to be healed. We know what the priorities are. We know where to start. Where there is purity, there is Your presence. And where there is Your presence, there is Your power. So we start at the right place. And I thank you that your servant Bob reminded us of this critical aspect of praying for healing. In Jesus' name we come before you as a people, laying our lives before You, asking for Your purification process, Your burning away of the dross from us . . . The sins and the impurities of our lives—we throw them out. We turn away from them. We repent. We walk away from them . . . We walk away from our sins. We walk in purity before you, Father, knowing that the effectual fervent prayer of a righteous church availeth much. In Jesus' Name. Amen.

What an anointed service! We were both deeply moved as we saw the repentance that God was bringing within our own church body.

Another poignant moment followed for Chuck and me as we saw Joe, teacher of the three-year-old Sunday school class, approach the microphone. This single man had such a tender heart for children and we had often told him how we looked forward to Sterling being in his class someday. Joe shared an encouraging verse of scripture and concluded with: "I just look forward to the day in less than three years that I'll be able to teach Heidi in Sunday school!"

Over the next moments we watched hands go up, committing to pray and fast for Heidi. I couldn't believe my eyes. There were so many hands raised! And yet, I could believe it. These were godly, precious people who had become like family to us during the short nine-year history of the church.

Pastor Travis closed the time of corporate prayer:

> Father, we continue to stand on the Word. We do not stand on our own feelings. We do not stand on what the doctor's report is. But we stand on the character and nature of Jesus Christ and His Words which last forever. Father, You said in Psalm 107 that you sent forth Your Word and You healed them. And You delivered Heidi Joy from destruction. Let her parents and Heidi Joy praise the Lord for the steadfast love of the Lord. And for the great and mighty things that He has done to bring rejoicing and joy and praise to His holy name. We pray Matthew chapter 8 that Jesus went around doing good and healing all who were diseased. And this was to fulfill the words of the prophet Isaiah, "He took their infirmities and He bore away their diseases."
>
> And, Father, may the peace that surpasses all understanding keep our hearts and our minds in Christ Jesus. Father, Chuck's and Vickie's hearts and minds. Would you keep them in You? We come against depression. We come against discouragement . . . a feeling of loss for Chuck and Vickie. Would you well them up . . . hold them up in your love. Surround Your arms around them. Protect and comfort them in Jesus' name. Father, in the midst of the battle, would you bring them joy? In the

midst of the struggle, would you bring them victory? In the middle of bad news, would Your good news come deep within their hearts? Would You sew the seeds of Your Word deep within their hearts right now? So, Father, as You lift up Chuck and Vickie, at the same time we are continuing to remain steadfast and claim Your Word and Your healing on little Heidi Joy. Now, Father, make her dynamic for You as You give her a new heart in Christ Jesus. Amen!

What a boost to our faith! To know that we were not standing alone! And yet what a contrast to what the day had held when we looked at Heidi's condition. What we had just viewed had taken place that morning. Why had Heidi gotten worse throughout the day? That's not the way prayer was supposed to work. It was confusing to say the least.

———— ⪢⪢⪢ ————

Monday afternoon as we sat by Heidi's bedside, I felt the weariness of the battle. We had been reading the Bible to her and singing to her for awhile. Chuck stepped out to the waiting room to make phone calls.

There was no music left within me. "Heidi, let's listen to Sandi Patti sing your song," I suggested, inserting the tape into the cassette player. I had been singing the first verse to her on each visit. The words to the second verse had slipped my mind, so it had been awhile since I had heard the tape. This time the prelude of Scripture did not sting. It ministered deeply to me:

> *You made my whole being;*
> *You formed me in my mother's body.*

You saw my bones being formed
as I took shape in my mother's body.
When I was put together there,
You saw my body as it was formed.
I praise You
because You made me
in an amazing and wonderful way.

I remembered questioning God seven months earlier. Was this really the verse for my child? I had wanted something more unique. Now I understood. It was perfect for Heidi and for our situation. God was not surprised by anything that was happening. He *knew* about her heart when He gave me those verses. That brought comfort.

Heidi briefly opened her eyes as Sandi began to sing. I think it was her way of letting me know that she noticed the difference between Mommy's voice and that of Sandi Patti. Smart girl!

I held her hand as we listened to the song. Unlike the night of her birth, this time I heard all of the words, *especially* the second verse:

Before you had a name or opened up your eyes
Or anyone could recognize your face,
You were being formed so delicate in size
Secluded in God's safe and hidden place.
With your little tiny hands and little tiny feet
And little eyes that shimmer like a pearl,
He breathed in you a song and to make it all complete
He brought the masterpiece into the world.

You are a masterpiece,
A new creation He has formed

And you're as soft and fresh as a snowy winter morn.
And I'm so glad that God has given you to me
Little Lamb of God
You are a masterpiece.

And now you're growing up, your life's a miracle
Every time I look at you, I stand in awe
Because I see in you a reflection of me.
And you'll always be my little Lamb from God
*And **as your life goes on each day,***
How I pray that you will see
Just how much your life has meant to me.
And I'm so proud of you
What else is there to say
Just be the masterpiece He created you to be.

You are a masterpiece,
A new creation He has formed
And you're as soft and fresh as a snowy winter morn.
And I'm so glad that God has given you to me
Little Lamb of God
You are a masterpiece. [1]

There it was! He had already told me what I needed to know about Heidi! It was right there in her song! The second verse said, "Now you're growing up, your life's a miracle!" That was my answer! God told me that she would grow up! He had given me the word long before I even knew I needed it. God would not tell me that she would grow up if she were going to die.

At that moment, I knew that Heidi would live. I didn't know how we were going to get from Point A "she's dying" to Point B "she's a miracle." But I knew God had given me my answer. She would live!

During those precious moments, I was given the gift of faith—my part in the battle plan. It was given much like a birthday gift that I would give to Sterling. He wouldn't have earned it. He wouldn't have to prove anything by it. It would simply be placed into his hands as a present chosen to be suitable for him by his mother who knows his needs.

And so it was with my gift of faith from God. I had done nothing to earn it. I had not wished it into being (although I would have if possible). I would not have to prove anything by it. It was simply placed in my hands as a gift chosen to be suitable for me by my heavenly Father who knows my needs.

What do you do when what you see with your eyes is so vastly different from what God has told you beforehand about the situation? I had two clear choices:

(1) To believe what I saw with my eyes and heard from a skilled medical community, or

(2) To believe what God had told me about her, months before her birth. I chose the latter.

No, I still didn't know "how" but I knew "what." My daughter was going to live and be a miracle. I knew that I knew that I knew. And no one could convince me otherwise. I had heard from God. I would speak what God said about her. I would expect what God said concerning her. I would focus on what God said about the circumstances until I saw the circumstances line up with His Word.

Chapter Five

How Do You Walk Out Your Faith?

When Chuck returned to the NICU, he found a different woman. The change in me was drastic. The numbness and fog had been replaced by determination.

Moments before, I had told Heidi the news with a conviction that I was speaking truth this time. "Heidi Joy, God says that you are a masterpiece. You *will* grow up. You are going to live and not die. So no matter what you hear anyone else say, you remember what God says about you. If what you hear doesn't line up with what God says, then don't receive it in your spirit or your body, honey. *He* says that your life will be a miracle. We're going to fight together. Don't give up.

"You *will* come off of this respirator. You will learn to breathe on your own because God has placed that knowledge within you. Life is going to get easier. It won't always be this hard. But for now, keep fighting. God is healing your heart. And there will be a day soon when it will work right."

Tears of pain were replaced by tears of joy as I told Chuck what had happened. I wanted to pick up Heidi and swing her around. But that would have to come later. Get rid of the tubes first.

Meanwhile, what was I to do differently? If I really believed that my daughter was going to live, how was I to walk out that faith now? I had heard of taking "steps of faith" all my life, but what were those "steps" in believing for the healing of a newborn? God had to show me.

That night as Chuck and I drove home on the deserted freeways of Fort Worth at midnight, I brought up the subject of breast feeding. It had come to mind several times throughout the afternoon. In the waiting room I had overheard a mother talking about pumping milk for her NICU baby. I had breast-fed Sterling as an infant, and we both felt it was the healthiest choice for our children. Heidi was still on total IV fluid feedings. There had been no mention of milk yet.

"Chuck, I think I'm supposed to pump breast milk for Heidi. Kind of like a step of faith that I believe she will be healed and need it. Also for her health," I ventured.

"How do you do that with Heidi on IVs?" he asked.

"There are electric breast pumps which can extract the milk. I heard one mother talking in the waiting room today. Evidently there is a private room on Side B of the NICU equipped with an electric pump for mothers to use. I could use that one while we're at the hospital and maybe we could rent one for home from a medical supply company," I explained.

"You don't have to do it if you feel like it's too much," he replied. "That would be a big commitment on your part. How long would it take each time? And how often would you need to pump?"

"It would probably take about twenty to twenty-five minutes each time. And I would need to pump every four hours to keep my milk supply going. My body will probably start producing milk within the next twenty-four hours, so we need to make a decision which way to go by that time. I'm surprised my milk isn't already in.

"The milk can be frozen for up to three months. But she'll be taking it from me long before then," I smiled. "I know it's a big commitment on my part. But there are two reasons I want to do it. The main reason is that I think it's one of the ways I'm supposed to walk out my faith. I believe that she will come off of the IVs and tubes and respirator, and need this milk to drink. We agree that it's the healthiest nutrition for her, so it's one of the few things I can do to contribute to her health.

"It will also keep me motivated to eat healthy and get plenty of rest. I was thinking about that earlier tonight. Neither of us can afford to let our bodies run down. Someone must be praying for our rest already, because I've been amazed at the quality of sleep for me. No nightmares! And these days have certainly had their share of nightmare-producing material. When my head hits the pillow, I'm able to go right to sleep. That's a blessing!"

"Well, you know I'll support you in this one hundred percent if you're up to doing it," he encouraged.

By noon the next day, there was an electric breast pump hooked up beside the recliner in our bedroom. Chuck had rented it from a local pharmacy. He wasn't wasting a minute. He was moving ahead in carrying out the battle plan. My body started producing milk that day as if on cue.

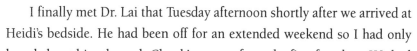

I finally met Dr. Lai that Tuesday afternoon shortly after we arrived at Heidi's bedside. He had been off for an extended weekend so I had only heard about him through Chuck's reports from the first few days. We had seen his partners daily over the weekend and on Monday.

Everything about Stephen Lai spoke precision—his appearance, his manner of speaking, even his walk. I liked the fact that the man checking out my daughter's heart was detail-oriented. He was of Chinese descent, speaking impeccable English, and immaculately dressed. His crisply starched blue and white striped shirt and perfectly-matched tie were part of an exquisite wardrobe which we would see in the days ahead. He was shorter than both of us, but I was intimidated by his clipped, authoritative manner of communicating. I could tell by his greeting to Chuck that the two of them already had a good working relationship.

He drew two diagrams for us, one of a normal heart and one showing Heidi's heart. What a contrast! It gave us a picture of the medical terms that were now becoming familiar to us—Ebstein's Anomaly, tricuspid valve, cardiomegaly, vastly enlarged right atrium.

In his diagram, her right atrium looked like an over-inflated balloon compared to her other three heart chambers. The bottom of that atrium extended far down into her right ventricle chamber. Where there should have been a tricuspid valve composed of three tissue flaps which met in a seal and then separated as they pumped the blood through the heart, there was only a gaping hole. Three pieces of tissue hung limply from that opening, barely fluttering. They didn't come close to sealing. They didn't even touch!

Rather than pumping forward through the heart and on out into the lungs and body, the blood was sloshing back into her right atrium. The regurgitation of the blood back into the atrium was what caused the sound of her loud heart murmur.

Dr. Lai's words were as to-the-point as his diagram. "Mr. and Mrs. Watson, Heidi was born in serious condition. She is now six days old, and we had hoped to see some improvement in her condition by this time. As you know, there has been *no* improvement. Her condition is deteriorating daily. We've already been forced to use prostaglandin. That is saved for last-resort measures. Our options are fewer every day."

"What are our options right now?" Chuck asked.

"Our goal is to wean her off the respirator while she's still on the prostaglandin. Then we'll try to wean the prostaglandin. But that has to happen soon. She cannot stay on this medication very long. We're hoping for a window of opportunity to get the respirator off. We don't have a lot of time to work with. And so far, time has not been in our favor," he explained. "Do you have any questions?"

I looked down at Heidi. Why did she have to hear all of this? *Remember, Heidi, don't receive that report. It's not what God says about you,* I pleaded inwardly.

Chuck spoke up, as if reading my thoughts. "Dr. Lai, there are a couple of requests we have. We appreciate the accuracy of your work and the information you bring to us. But if it is of a negative nature—bad news—we request that you not tell us within Heidi's hearing. We'll be glad to step to the other side of the room or out in the hallway, whatever works best for you. We just don't want negative reports given at her bedside."

Of course that meant all medical reports right now. There had been no good news medically since her birth. The confused look on Dr. Lai's face followed by his brief, "Okay," told me that he was probably thinking we were nuts.

I wanted to step in and explain. Explain ourselves and our Christian belief. Explain what God had told me about Heidi before her birth. Explain that she was going to be healed. Explain that we really did understand that she was a newborn. That she didn't have a grasp of the English language yet. That she didn't comprehend what he was saying. But that her spirit was receiving those words, thus affecting her body.

Chuck wisely moved on, unmoved by what Dr. Lai might think of us or our request. "Also, Vickie is pumping breast milk for Heidi and freezing it. We wanted you to know that it will be available as soon as she can nurse or take bottles. We prefer that she have breast milk rather than formula when that time comes."

I could just imagine his thoughts as he quickly ended the conversation and left the room—*These parents are totally out of touch with reality. I tell them that their daughter has gone downhill from being in serious condition, and their response? Don't talk negatively around her. And by the way, we have breast milk ready for her feedings. Didn't they hear anything I said? These parents are as rare as their daughter's heart defect!*

Chuck's voice jolted me back to the present. "Vickie, you're worried about what Dr. Lai is thinking of us right now, aren't you?" He knew me well. "Don't worry about it! Our job as parents is to speak up for Heidi's needs. We are her voice. Don't expect the doctors or nurses to understand where we're coming from. We all make up a team working together on Heidi's behalf."

Once again I clearly saw Chuck's gifting from God for this battle. He had the big picture in focus as well as the details of her care. Over the next few weeks, God gave me four more specific ways to "walk out my faith."

One morning, I tackled the growing stack of mail on our dining room table. We daily pulled out the cards and letters of encouragement to read on the way to the hospital, stacking the "regular" items aside for later. By the size of the stack I knew we would soon need to go through the mail or get a larger table.

Maybe there were some personal notes we had missed! So far there had been only bills and junk mail and requests for donations.

I opened yet another envelope addressed "to the parents of Baby Watson." How do all those companies get your address when you have a baby? No, we didn't want diaper service. No, we didn't want personalized baby shoes. No, we didn't need our baby's picture taken. No, we didn't want life insurance for our baby.

Wait a minute! The advertisement said we could purchase a six month $10,000 policy for $1.00. No questions asked. Wouldn't that be using wisdom? There's nothing wrong with life insurance. We had coverage on Chuck and me. I vaguely remembered a policy covering our children as a part of Chuck's benefit package at American Airlines.

Had we purchased extra coverage for Sterling? No. But Heidi's situation was different. What if we carried the policy for just six months and then dropped it? No harm done. Only a dollar out of our pockets. By then, we would certainly know where Heidi stood.

"Do you believe that I'm going to heal Heidi?" came the gentle nudge of the Holy Spirit.

"Of course I do. We just don't want to be unwise," I reasoned.

"Do you *really* believe that I'm going to heal her?" The nudging was stronger. "Then stop trying to cover yourself in case it doesn't happen. Don't waste your dollar!"

I tore up the ad, just in case I might be tempted to dig it out later. As the pieces floated downward into the trash can, I watched perplexed. This walking out your faith thing was certainly not as "spiritual" as I had expected.

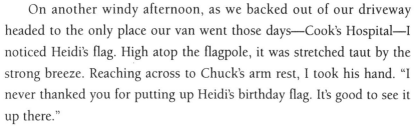

On another windy afternoon, as we backed out of our driveway headed to the only place our van went those days—Cook's Hospital—I noticed Heidi's flag. High atop the flagpole, it was stretched taut by the strong breeze. Reaching across to Chuck's arm rest, I took his hand. "I never thanked you for putting up Heidi's birthday flag. It's good to see it up there."

"I'm glad," he responded. "You hadn't mentioned it, so I wasn't sure. I thought maybe it was too painful for you. Sterling and I put it up on Saturday morning just before I came to pick you up at HEB Hospital."

"Thanks. It *was* painful the first day we came home without her. A part of me wanted to rip it down. My mind had painted a picture of the moment we would bring her home. And I had done everything possible to get the setting ready. The pansies. The flag. The cradle. I never dreamed Heidi would be the missing element," I tearfully confessed.

We were getting used to the constant presence of tears. A sound, a word, even a flag could usher them in. It didn't take much!

"I'm really glad you raised her flag," I continued. "It's a tangible reminder here at home that she's a part of us. I like that. It's also an announcement to the neighborhood. We have a daughter! Yes, she's fighting for her life. But we have a new daughter! That's something to celebrate! A new life!

"You know what? Don't take the flag down at the end of her first week. The idea just came to me. We're supposed to fly her flag until the day she comes home from the hospital—whether that's tomorrow or another week or two."

There it was. Step number three in the walk of faith.

One morning as Chuck, Sterling, and I dressed for the day, I approached Chuck with another of my ideas. It was starting to dawn on me that some of these "ideas" were promptings of the Holy Spirit.

"Honey, I've been thinking about recording a cassette tape for Heidi, for the times when I'm not there and for my less faith-filled moments. I would read the scripture verses God has given us for her, sing to her, and tell her about us. About what life will be like in our family, and the things we are going to do as she grows up. It would be another way to be sure she's daily hearing what God says about her. What do you think?"

The words were barely out of my mouth before he handed me the tape recorder and a blank tape. "Go for it!" he encouraged. "Why don't you do it in your closet? It's the quietest place with no interruptions."

"You mean right now?"

"Sure. You're supposed to do it. Now is the best time. I'll watch Sterling and keep things as quiet as possible."

After seven and one-half years of marriage, I should have known that Chuck would have me doing it within minutes. He's a man of action. I appreciate that. He moves us forward, although at times I'm panting to keep up.

My large walk-in closet was the perfect spot. Cassette recorder, blank tape, and Bible. I was ready to go within minutes.

For the first few minutes, I shared with Heidi how much we loved her and then read her verses from Psalm 139. I decided to double-check the sound on the recorder, just to be certain everything was working. As I played it back, I heard a tired, depressing voice. Who would dream of listening to this for encouragement?

Start over. Take two. Remember, this is to impart hope to Heidi's spirit, not to let her know how depressed her mother's voice can sound. This time it was better.

> Heidi, this is Mommy. I'm going to read to you what God has said about you. He gave me this first scripture while you were still in my tummy, before I had ever seen you. God says that He formed your inward parts; He did weave you in my womb. We give thanks to God, because you are fearfully and wonderfully made. Wonderful are God's works, and my soul and your soul knows it very well. Your frame was not hidden from God, when you were made in secret, and skillfully wrought in the depths of the earth. God's eyes saw your unformed substance; and in God's book they were all written, the days that were ordained for you, when as yet there was not one of them. That's what God says about you.
>
> He says He has covered your head in the day of battle. God the Lord is the strength of my salvation. And God is your strength, Heidi.

The Lord sustains all who fall, and raises up all who are bowed down. The eyes of all look to God, and He gives them their food in due time. Thou dost open Thy hand and satisfy the desire of every living thing. The Lord is righteous in all His ways and kind in all His deeds. He is near to all who call upon Him, to all who call upon Him in truth.

Do not trust in princes, in mortal man, in whom there is no salvation. How blessed is he whose help is the God of Jacob. And that's who is your help, Heidi Joy. The God of Jacob. How blessed is he whose hope is in the Lord his God.

For He has strengthened the bars of your gates. That's your heart valves. He has blessed your sons within you. That's the children that are to come to you because you are to be a joyful mother of children. He makes peace in your borders. He has given peace to your spirit and continues to do so. He satisfies you with the finest of the wheat.

The Lord will accomplish what concerns you. Though you walk in the midst of trouble, the Lord will revive you. He is the one reviving you now, Heidi Joy. Spirit of God, revive Heidi Joy's spirit and her soul and her body. He stretches forth His hand against the wrath of your enemies, and His right hand has saved you, Heidi. The Lord has accomplished what concerns you. His loving-kindness is everlasting. He has not forsaken the works of His hands, Heidi. Not at all.

How precious is Thy loving-kindness, O God! And the children of men take refuge in the shadow of Thy wings. Heidi, God is holding you in the shadow of His wings right now. You are in His refuge. You drink your fill of the abundance of His house. And He gives you to drink of the river of His delights. You are drinking from His delights, and that's health and healing. For with God is the fountain of life and He has flowed that fountain over you, Heidi Joy. Over your body, your heart, your lungs, over every working system within your body. He has flowed over that with the fountain of life.

In Thy light we see light. Heidi, our light is coming from God.

The Lord is your shepherd, Heidi Joy. You shall not want. He makes you to lie down in green pastures. He leads you beside quiet waters. He restores and revives your soul. He restores your body. He restores your mind. He guides you in the paths of righteousness for His name's sake and for His glory. Even though you have walked through the valley of the shadow of death, we fear no evil. For God has been and is and continues to be with you. His rod and His staff—they are your comfort. He has prepared a table before you in the presence of your enemies. And He has anointed your head with oil. Your cup overflows, Heidi. Surely His goodness and loving-kindness shall follow you all the days of your life. And you will dwell in the house of the Lord forever. Where it talks about God preparing a table before you in the presence of your enemies—it means that God as a gracious host has provided all that you need. He has provided it for you. (Footnote from *The Ryrie Study Bible* © 1976, 1978 by The Moody Bible Institute of Chicago)

Thus saith the Lord God unto your bones, "Behold, I will cause breath to enter into you and you shall live, Heidi." Know that in your spirit, honey. God says, "**You shall live**" because He has caused the breath to enter into your bones and He speaks life to you.

Because you relied on the Lord, He delivered your enemies into your hand. For the eyes of the Lord move to and fro throughout the earth that He may strongly support those whose heart is completely His. And, Heidi, we confess as we stand before God, that we can do nothing of our own accord. But we look to God, and we look at what He says about you. And that's what we stand on, honey, and that's stronger than what any man can say or do. And our heart is completely God's, as best as we know. We continue to plead for His mercy. And He says that He looks to and fro throughout the earth, that He may strongly support those whose heart is completely His. We have also given Him your heart, Heidi. Your heart is in God's hands, honey.

Those who wait for the Lord, they will inherit the land. Yet a little while and the wicked man will be no more. And you will look carefully for his place, and he will not be there. But the humble will inherit the land, and will delight themselves in abundant prosperity. God has for you, Heidi, an abundance of peace and truth. Peace over your spirit, honey. And the truth is the word of God. May your spirit not receive anything that doesn't line up with the word of God—with what God says about you, Heidi.

Mark the blameless man, and behold the upright;

for the man of peace will have a posterity. But transgressors will be altogether destroyed. The posterity of the wicked will be cut off. But the salvation of the righteous is from the Lord. The Lord God is who has brought your salvation, honey. He is your healer and He has done it. By His stripes you have been healed. The salvation of the righteous is from the Lord. He is your strength in time of trouble. And the Lord helps you and delivers you. He delivers you from the wicked and saves you, because we take refuge in Him. We take refuge in the Lord God, Heidi. (Psalm 139:13-16; 140:7; 145:14-18; 146:3,5; 147:13-14; 138:7-8; 36:7-9; 23:1-6; Ezekiel 37:5; II Chronicles 16:8-9; Psalm 37:9-11, 37-40 NASB)

There were many other things I wanted to share with her. But it was time to head to the hospital. I would tell Heidi more later. For now, it was a start.

Step number five proved to be just as "unspiritual" as the others. A week later, Chuck and I were headed out the back door on our daily trek to the hospital, when Mother stopped us. She had just awakened from one of her catnaps throughout the day, still trying to adjust to being up all night. She and Grandma Watson were now starting their "Sterling" shift. We had already kissed him good-bye and were crossing the back patio when Mother called to us. "Is there anything I can do for you today, Vickie? Besides changing your sheets, that is!"

We both laughed. Some household chores had been delayed over the past weeks while others had been *well* cared for. We had discovered in conversation that morning that our bedroom sheets had been changed three times within the past four days. Once by Mother and twice by telephone volunteers. Our needs were certainly being met abundantly!

"There is one thing I would love to have done, if you get a chance," I recalled. "Upstairs on the floor in Sterling's closet are two stacks of baby clothes. One stack has a note saying 'Wash if it's a boy.' The other says, 'Wash if it's a girl.' Would you wash the girl clothes and put them on the changing table in our bedroom with the other clean baby things?"

She nodded without a word. It was several days later before she brought up the subject again. "I washed those clothes for you. I have them folded and ready upstairs."

"Thanks," I replied. "When you get a chance, would you put them on the changing table in our bedroom? I want everything to be ready when Heidi comes home."

Again she nodded wordlessly. It was months later when Mother confided that it was the most difficult thing she had ever done for me. To bring those frilly dresses, lacy socks, and ruffled play suits to my bedroom where I would see them daily, while it still appeared that Heidi would never wear them—that was tough!

I realized that our parents were experiencing this crisis at two levels. One as a grandparent aching for their grandchild. Another as a parent watching their child hurt. The experience was challenging and growing all of us in different ways.

The baby clothes episode? It was a step of faith. I was to prepare for her homecoming.

——————— ⋙~ ———————

Another step of faith also involved clothing. Nothing had changed about Heidi's condition. She had continued her downward decline.

Adrienne called one morning to get an update from the phone volunteer. She was a close friend, a mother of five, a Bible study comrade, and a woman who sought God's perspective in everything. Ours was one of those rare relationships where you're both good for each other.

"Vickie, I've got a question for you. I think I know the answer, but I promised I would ask. Connie from your care group called. She has been sensing that she is to make a christening gown for Heidi. She's aware of the latest reports, but said that she just can't get it off her mind. But she doesn't want to do it if it's too painful for you. What do you think?"

Finally, a question with an easy answer. "Yes! Tell her to send it over as soon as it's finished. It will hang in our bedroom until the day she wears it at her dedication. Yes, go for it!" I almost shouted into the phone.

If Connie made it, it would be beautiful. She was an accomplished seamstress. But I was most excited that God was prompting someone else with steps of faith headed in the same direction as mine.

Heidi had been given one soft white dress with tiny pink rosebuds from Doug and Nancy on the night of her birth. Since that time, many stuffed animals, flowers, fruit baskets, and cards of encouragement had arrived. But it hit me after I hung up the phone. There were no gifts of clothes. People don't give clothes to a baby who is dying. That would be too painful later on when the baby was gone. No, anything but clothes for a baby who won't make it.

So I was even more excited about Connie's offer. To me, it was a sign that she believed Heidi would live to wear that dress.

When she brought it over several days later, it was beautiful. I discovered it hanging in the living room as Chuck and I tiptoed in one midnight. Snow white with tiny tucks across the bodice. Daintily puffed sleeves topped with a white rose and bow. The three-foot skirt ended in three rows of scalloped lace. A single miniature red rose with red and white ribbons cascading downward accented the bodice. The matching bonnet was adorned with the same lace. It tied under the chin with white ribbon attached by two white roses. It was precious.

The only thing I would change would be the red rose and red ribbon. Pink was Heidi's color in my mind. I would switch that later. For now, it belonged in our bedroom, hanging from the heart-shaped shelf on the wall beside the changing table. I fell asleep that night gazing at it from my pillow.

If I really believed my daughter was going to live, what was I to do differently? Pump breast milk. Don't purchase extra life insurance—even for one dollar. Fly Heidi's birthday flag until she came home. Wash the dresses. Say yes to the offer of a christening gown.

I've heard of "steps of faith" all my life, but I didn't know they would be so practical—so ordinary. Spiritual? They became *very* spiritual when they involved obeying the prompting of the Holy Spirit.

Chapter Six

WHAT DO YOU DO WITH THANKSGIVING DAY?

Early Tuesday afternoon, our friend Gloria telephoned from Waco, Texas. "What are you doing for Thanksgiving dinner?" she asked, after getting a Heidi update.

It was my first recollection since Heidi's birth that there *was* a Thanksgiving Day that week. Heidi would be one week old on Thanksgiving Day! Her condition? Not good.

The doctors' reports:

> Nothing has gone as we had hoped. She was born in critical condition and is worsening daily. "Massive cardiomegaly (enlarged heart) . . . tricuspid valve very incompetent" . . . tried to wean from prostaglandin . . . "baby began dropping oxygen saturation levels to 50's, became dusky so prostaglandin restarted . . . prognosis remains guarded."

Grandma Boone's journal:

> On Monday and Tuesday Heidi was really low. They tried to bring her off the respirator, but couldn't . . . She got blue, had chills and fever . . . was in much stress and pain . . . morphine . . . very labored breathing . . . body very puffy . . . gave her Lasix to hopefully get rid of fluid.

But I knew what we were to do. Celebrate a day of Thanksgiving! Of all years, we especially had something to be grateful for this year—Heidi was alive!

"Vickie, are you still there?" Gloria's voice interrupted my thoughts.

"Yes, I'm here. We want to *celebrate* on Thanksgiving. To give thanks that Heidi is alive," I answered confidently.

"Then I have a plan." Gloria is a female version of Chuck in many ways. Lover of people. Has a plan, along with the energy to make it happen. Welcomes new experiences. A dear friend to both Chuck and me. When she had been a bridesmaid in our wedding at the age of fifty-three, we had to keep reminding her not to dance down the aisle!

"Here's my plan." I could hear the excitement building in her voice. "I'll cook a turkey dinner for your household—whoever that includes this week. Thursday morning, I'll drive over from Waco, and we'll have Thanksgiving dinner together. I'd love to do this for your family. What do you think?"

"Well, I think it's the first time we've ever had Thanksgiving dinner catered ninety miles, but it sounds great! What do we need to do here?"

"Nothing. Just take care of Heidi. Get some rest. And I'll see you all Thursday morning! My Sunday school class and I are praying," she reminded me.

It was set. We would celebrate Thanksgiving. The timing seemed right.

Glen and Bronwyn, a couple from our church, stayed with Heidi through the night on Wednesday to give the grandmothers some sleep. Thursday morning, Grandmas Boone and Watson were at the hospital from seven thirty until noon when they joined us for dinner.

As we gathered around our dining room table, there was a mixture of emotions. Some wondered how I could go through the motions of a holiday with my baby dying. But these were not empty motions. It was the truest expression of gratitude I had ever known on Thanksgiving Day. I was grateful for the fact that my daughter was alive at that moment, and also overwhelmed by the support given to us that week. The prayers, the food, the telephone volunteers, the cards. The constant ringing of the phone (at least fifty calls per day) with calls from all over the world signaled that people were praying.

Even this feast before us was evidence of God's provision for us through family and friends. I wasn't sure how Gloria had transported it in her car. There was turkey with dressing, mashed potatoes and gravy, green beans, sweet potato casserole, cranberry sauce, waldorf salad, homemade rolls, and pumpkin pies.

The long dining room table was draped with a soft blue tablecloth and set with our wedding china—cream colored plates accented with tiny pink and blue flowers. The faces lining the table were dear ones. Chuck, Sterling, Grandma Watson, Grandma Boone, Gloria, and Rose Annette with six-year-old Jessica and eight-year-old Jeremy.

At the hospital were Grandpa Boone and Bryan. It didn't hit me until that moment that they were willing to give up the holiday dinner with their families. They had agreed to delay their feasting until three o'clock when Chuck and I would go to Heidi.

Grandma Watson and Gloria had their memories of earlier holidays with their husbands who were now in heaven. As we lingered over pumpkin pie and coffee, my thoughts turned toward our family's Thanksgiving mealtime tradition. "Let's share what we're most grateful for from the past year."

As we each spoke, Jeremy and Jessica seemed puzzled at times by this one-minute-laughing and the-next-minute-crying group of adults.

Sterling didn't care whether we laughed or cried. He was happy to be with his cousins.

It was finally my turn. "The last week has been so full of negative reports that I have to verbalize my gratitude for the good things. There *are* many blessings in my life. Number one for me is obvious—that Heidi Joy is alive today. And I'm grateful to be the wife of Chuck and the mother of Sterling and Heidi," I concluded tearfully.

The privilege of being a wife and mother would always be special to me. Since Chuck and I had not married until two months before my thirtieth birthday, there had been years of doubting that I would ever marry.

And when we had started discussing marriage, Chuck had surprised me with the news that he did not feel we were to have children. I hadn't expected this from a man who dearly loved little ones. He had often kept a set of single-parent three-year-old twins on weekends while their mother worked. Chuck felt that we were to give our time and energy to helping children from single-parent homes, rather than having children of our own.

After praying and processing his idea for several weeks, I came to a comfortable conclusion. "Chuck, I know you are the man God has provided for me. I have no doubts about that. I had always assumed that if I married I would have children, but I had no guarantee that I would ever marry. I accept your plan to have no children and agree to never bring up the subject again," I had told him.

"Oh, no," he quickly interjected. "I'm not asking you to do that."

"I know," I replied. "But this is a commitment I need to make to myself at this point. I don't want to be trying to talk you into having children some day down the road. Or pointing out new babies in hopes that you will change your mind. If you should ever change your mind, I want it to be because God has changed your heart about the matter, not that Vickie has manipulated the circumstances. So I need to make that commitment to you as a safeguard for both of us. And no one needs to know whose idea it was. This is a joint decision."

Three and one-half years into our marriage, Mike (Adrienne's husband) had questioned Chuck rather pointedly on the subject of our not having children. His challenge to Chuck was strong. "More than anyone I know, you have given God total control of every area of your life, except one—that of children. And in that area you have chosen to make the decision without His input. The Bible says that children are a blessing from the Lord and that God opens and closes the womb. I challenge you to stop using birth control and allow God to make that decision. If it is truly His desire that you have no children, He can close the womb."

Chuck shared the conversation with me. Over the next year, he processed Mike's challenge and on January 1 shared with me where he felt God was leading us. "I think we are to stop using birth control, Vickie, and see if God chooses to open or close your womb. It's no guarantee that we'll get pregnant, you know. I just don't want you to get your hopes up that we will have a baby, because that still may not happen."

I was thrilled. Over the last several years, my maternal instincts had awakened as I had watched friends having babies. My commitment to keep quiet about the subject had led me to pray that God would either change my desires or Chuck's heart. It had been a powerful lesson for me—seeing God's hand rather than Vickie's mouth at work. It had also been a potent reminder of what God does when I ask Him to show my husband the plan for our family, rather than me telling friends my desires for our family.

Five months later we were pregnant with Sterling. So the opportunity to be a wife and mother would always be a special reminder of God's provision for me, at Thanksgiving, as well as throughout the year.

That Thanksgiving afternoon Sterling was allowed a short visit into the NICU to meet his sister. It was the first time the four of us had been together. He seemed less startled by the tubes and wires than many adults. This was his sister "Hi-he" whom he had heard about so much. He enjoyed kissing her fingers.

That evening I made my first journal entry since her birth. It was in the form of a letter:

> Dear Heidi Joy, You are one week old today. Thank you, Lord! The last week has been the most painful and yet most hopeful of our lives.
>
> You are now in critical condition in the NICU at Cook's Hospital. That's what we see with our physical eyes. We have seen you work hard to breathe, tremble for hours from the medicine, scream in pain without making a sound (because of the tubes in your throat), gag on the respirator tubes, swell from fluid, go through a medical procedure to place a central line for IVs when your other veins had collapsed. That's what we've seen with our physical eyes.
>
> We've sat by your bedside and held your hand, cried, read scripture, sang songs. There have been moments of faith—knowing what God says about you, even though things physically look so different. And there have been the moments when our pain was unbearable as we watched your pain—so we just sat with you and cried.

My journal entry ended abruptly with wet smudges on the paper. Throughout that holiday weekend, Heidi's condition continued its downward slide.

My journal on Friday reflected Dr. Lai's report:

> **Dr. Lai's report:** Blood flowing forward from heart to lungs—still not enough.
>
> **GOD'S report:** "For He has strengthened the bars of your gates" (valves). (Psalm 147:13, NASB)
>
> **Dr. Lai's report:** She's hungry—being given nutrients to sustain but not enough to satisfy.
>
> **GOD'S report:** "He satisfies you with the finest of the wheat." (Psalm 147:14, NASB)
>
> **Dr. Lai's report:** Lungs still stiff.
>
> **GOD'S report:** "Thus saith the Lord God unto these bones, 'Behold, I will cause breath to enter into you, and ye shall live.'" (Ezekiel 37:5, KJV)
>
> **Dr. Lai's report:** Give it at least another week; won't attempt to stop prostaglandin or respirator until first of next week.
>
> **GOD'S report:** Word of knowledge through nephew Jeremy—WAIT! I think God is saying to be patient.
>
> **Dr. Lai's report:** Artificial bridge vessel (shunt) to get blood to lungs is no longer a good option.
>
> **GOD'S report:** "The Lord will accomplish what concerns me; Thy loving-kindness, O Lord, is everlasting; Do not forsake the works of Thy hands." (Psalm 138:8, NASB)

The medical report was in no way encouraging. But I certainly liked what God was saying. It was amazing to see how He had an answer for each segment of the medical report. I just wanted to *see* His solutions with my eyes.

————— ➤ —————

As I settled into our bedroom recliner at one-thirty a.m. to read the cards from that day's mail, I opened a gem from a lady in our church—another Vicki. She wrote: "Probably you know that Heidi means 'battle maiden' in German (according to the *Names for Boys and Girls* booklet from HEB). Indeed she is."

So that's why we named her "Heidi." Chuck and I wept over the card. We were learning that we don't always understand *why* God directs in a certain way. The important thing is our obedience.

————— ➤ —————

On Saturday God gave me one more unexpected Thanksgiving holiday gift. It was a day of questioning for me, as reflected in my journal:

> Are we doing enough? Why don't we physically *see* Heidi's healing? What are we supposed to do as we sit by her bedside? Is our weariness transferring to her spirit? Is it because we're so weary that we're not praying and reading the Word over her continually? Or is it okay to wait—since we've already asked Him?
> Answer: Lamentations 3:19-26
> ". . . This I recall to my mind,
> Therefore I have *hope*.
> The Lord's loving-kindnesses indeed never cease,
> For His compassions never fail . . .
> The Lord is good to those who wait for Him,

to the person who seeks Him.
It is good that he waits silently
For the salvation of the Lord." (NASB)

It was okay to wait silently.

Just before we were to leave late that night, Chuck approached the nurse with a question that surprised both the nurse and me. "When can my wife hold Heidi?"

Startled, the nurse went to check with the doctor on duty. I couldn't believe her response when she returned. "I think we could try it right now. We don't usually allow babies on respirators to be held because of the difficulty in moving them with the tube down their throat. But the doctor thinks it's worth a try."

We later learned the true reason I was allowed to hold her. Because they believed her to be dying, they granted our request. It was one of the few things they could do for us.

I had yearned for this moment. Dreamed of it. Longed for it over the past ten days. And it was suddenly here. This was too good to be true. Yet I heard myself saying, "If this doesn't work, please put her right back in the bed. I don't want to cause her any extra pain. Just be ready to take her if she starts crying."

It took five minutes for the three of us to transfer her from the bed to my arms. The maze of wires and tubes snaked from her bed to my chair. Within minutes of wrapping her in the blanket in my arms, she fell asleep. Her oxygen saturation levels and her heart beat improved immediately.

"It's working!" exclaimed Chuck. "That's exactly what I expected!"

My journal recorded the event:

11:30 p.m. on 11/30/91—I held Heidi for the first

time . . . 30-45 minutes . . . she's a wonderful cuddler . . . went to sleep in my arms. It's the first thing that has felt normal since her birth. It was wonderful! Can't wait for Chuck to hold her too.

Chapter Seven

How Much Have You Thought About Her Dying?

By the first week of December, we were starting to settle into a routine of sorts. Chuck would work at American Airlines each morning and into the afternoon. His boss was gracious in her directive to "do what must be done." Each day we headed to the hospital by mid-afternoon. He would finish any paperwork at Heidi's bedside and make calls from the waiting room.

Every few days, Gaylene brought Chuck's administrative church work to our home or the hospital. They talked daily by phone. Gaylene had been a dear friend for seven years. She had directed our wedding. She had lived with us two summers while volunteering at the church during her summer vacation from teaching. We had walked with her through the tragic death of her brother in a car accident. We had been attendants in her wedding to Dave. She now was employed as Chuck's assistant at the church. Her efficient organization, coupled with her love for us, was a godsend. Chuck tackled his church paper stack during the evening hours at the hospital.

The first week of December brought further medical complications. The previous week's medical procedure had been to implant a central line for IVs. All other veins had collapsed by now. They had to have an IV line available at all times to administer emergency medications in case her heart stopped.

Monday, December 2 — My journal reflected our medical conference that afternoon:

> **Dr. Smith's report:** Right upper lobe of lungs not expanding as should; heart probably pressing on it; lungs partially collapsed; heart ductus still open; some forward flow from right side of heart, but no more; no guarantee could make things better with shunt surgery.
>
> **GOD'S report:** He is the mender of hearts (word Laura received the day Heidi was born).
>
> **Dr. Smith's report:** Most concerning thing for him— seeing no improvement.
>
> **GOD'S report:** Word through Pastor Travis; has been interceding extensively for Heidi; yesterday afternoon felt God saying that we have interceded and asked; next part is to move into praise; praise infused into her spirit will come against bad effects of morphine, etc.; "For we are powerless before this great multitude who are coming against us; nor do we know what to do, but our eyes are on Thee." II Chronicles 20:12b (NASB)
>
> **Dr. Smith's report:** Two goals—off respirator and prostaglandin.
>
> **GOD'S report:** "Because you relied on the Lord, He delivered them into your hand. For the eyes of the Lord move to and fro throughout the earth that He may strongly support those whose heart is completely His." (II Chronicles 16:8b-9a, NASB)

Pastor Travis' words had deeply ministered to me on Sunday night as he had walked through the story of Jehoshaphat's victory in II Chronicles 20. I underlined many phrases as we read it together by Heidi's bedside that evening:

> "*A great multitude is coming against you* from beyond
> the sea" . . . Jehoshaphat was afraid and turned his atten-
> tion to seek the Lord; and proclaimed a fast . . . Judah
> gathered together to *seek help from the Lord . . . Power
> and might are in Thy hand* so that no one can stand
> against Thee . . . we will stand before this house and
> before Thee . . . and cry to Thee in our distress, and
> Thou wilt hear and deliver us . . . *we are powerless* before
> this great multitude who are coming against us; *nor do
> we know what to do, but our eyes are on Thee* . . . all Judah
> was standing before the Lord . . . *Do not fear or be dis-
> mayed* because of this great multitude, *for the battle is not
> yours but God's* . . . go down against them . . . You need
> not fight in this battle; station yourselves, *stand and see
> the salvation of the Lord on your behalf* . . . Do not fear or
> be dismayed; tomorrow go out to face them, for *the Lord
> is with you* . . . the inhabitants of Jerusalem fell down
> before the Lord, worshipping the Lord . . . stood up to
> praise the Lord God of Israel, with a very loud voice . . .
> Listen to me, O Judah and inhabitants of Jerusalem, *put
> your trust in the Lord your God*, and you will be estab-
> lished. Put your trust in His prophets and succeed . . . he
> appointed those who sang to the Lord and those who
> praised Him in holy attire, as they went out before the
> army and said, "Give thanks to the Lord, for His loving-
> kindness is everlasting." And *when they began singing
> and praising, the Lord set ambushes* against the sons of
> Ammon . . . destroying them completely . . . no one had

escaped. And when Jehoshaphat and his people came to
take their spoil [the good that God would bring out of
this], they found much . . . goods, garments, and valu-
able things, . . . more than they could carry . . . they
assembled in the *valley of Beracah [blessing]*, for there
they blessed the Lord . . . returning to Jerusalem with
joy, for the Lord had made them to rejoice over their
enemies . . . So *the kingdom of Jehoshaphat was at peace*,
for his God gave him rest on all sides. (II Chronicles 20,
NASB)

Pastor Travis' visit that night was an interesting study in contrasts.
This tall, gentle-spirited, rancher-turned-minister had walked through
deep waters in his almost fifty years. His understanding of healing came
from a personal battle with life-threatening lupus. Without God's miraculous touch, he would not have been alive to minister to us that evening.
The tender shepherd's-heart part of him was weeping and hurting with
us. The I've-heard-from-God part of him was jumping up and down
saying, "I've been called to praise God for what He is doing in Heidi's
behalf. Yippee!"

The joy within him kept bursting through as he would apologetically
say, "I do recognize how painful this must be right now watching her. But
I've been called to praise on her behalf. I hope that doesn't seem calloused
to you."

"Oh, no," I assured him. "You praise God. It certainly sounds better
than what we've heard today."

Here was another nugget about faith. I was starting to see how much
our obedience to the Holy Spirit's nudging affects what He is doing in
someone else's life. Pastor Travis' willingness to say he would be praising
God while looking at a baby whose condition worsened daily. Connie's

obedience in asking to make a christening gown for a baby who appeared to be dying. Their offers could have been rebuffed by us and labeled "insensitive." Yet these were the very things that powerfully ministered to us. Our responsibility is obedience, not interpretation.

I also received a note that day from six-and-one-half-year-old Jessica who had been praying daily for her cousin.

> I love you, Heidey. Jessica. Decimber the first 1991.
> Dear Ant Vicky. I hope Heidey is better soon. it has been
> a long time since she hasint come home. I hope that she
> will come home soon. I miss you Ant Vicky.

Beneath the writing was a drawing labeled "a newborn baby." Yes, Jessica, it seems like a long time to me too.

Grandma Boone's journal reflected the wee hours of that night:

> Heidi had a bad night . . . At 1:00 a.m. they gave her
> morphine. From 12:30 until 2:00 she was breathing
> hard and purple and crying . . . I thought we were going
> to lose her . . . Her IV line closed up for the third time . . .
> Nurses really were worried and worked with her. After
> morphine and increased respirator rate she settled
> down about 2:30 a.m. and rested . . . About 4:00 a.m.
> she had another bad spell when they tried to draw blood
> for blood gases . . . turned purple . . . Her color really
> looks bad.

Tuesday, December 3 — Mid-morning Grandpa Boone called from the hospital to say that Heidi was much worse. The prayer chain was alerted.

Dr. Lai's written report that morning stated: "Not as clinically stable today . . . follow closely." When Chuck and I arrived at the hospital that afternoon, he once again walked us through the details of her worsening condition.

I escaped as quickly as possible with the excuse of pumping breast milk. I wanted to scream at him, *Don't rob me of my picture of Heidi. She will be healed and live to the glory of God! If your report doesn't match that, then don't tell me.*

Chuck could fill me in later on the rest of their conversation, but I didn't want to hear it right then. I welcomed the quiet seclusion of the pumping room. At least I wouldn't be interrupted there with more bad news.

Fifteen minutes later, the door burst open as I grabbed for a blanket to cover myself. Dr. Lai and Chuck stood breathless before me, obviously shaken. "Mrs. Watson, we have to talk. Heidi's heart stopped and we almost lost her. It's time to talk candidly. I'll meet you in the conference room in five minutes."

As Dr. Lai left the room, Chuck stood at my side trembling, white as a sheet. He tearfully replayed the last ten minutes for me. "Vickie, we were at her bedside, and Dr. Lai was showing me her heart on the sonogram. Our nurse was also there. Right in the middle of his explanation, Dr. Lai saw her heart stop beating on the sonogram. Her oxygen saturation level dropped to one and her pulse went to forty-eight. Monitors were shrieking. Staff came running to help. Dr. Lai administered heart compressions. They kicked me out of the room then. It was horrible," he sobbed. I sat numbly listening.

"They brought me back in after what seemed like an eternity. Dr. Lai told me what had happened. Dr. Turbeville had pulled out the respirator tube and put in a new one. It was four minutes before they had her breathing again. She almost died, Vickie! I thought we had lost her! It might have been too late if Dr. Lai had not been standing right there!"

Chuck concluded in tears. The visual images were still replaying through his mind. "We almost lost her!" he repeated.

My mind was blank. "Let's go talk to Dr. Lai," I numbly suggested, putting away the breast pump and storing the milk in the refrigerator. The sight of the rows of tiny milk bottles with "Heidi Joy Watson" labels stabbed at me. Then the thoughts came—*So, mighty woman of faith, you're the one who has pumped all of this milk for your baby. Her heart stopped while you were pumping it. Don't you think this is a waste of time? Give it up! You have enough on you already. Can't you see what's ahead? And this meeting with Dr. Lai. Your daughter was in cardiac arrest. How much more candid can you get? He has told you that she's worse every day. You know they think you're totally out to lunch. Out of touch with reality. Give up on this faith stuff and read the handwriting on the wall. Your child is dying. Don't you get it?* The Accuser was working full time.

Our meeting with Dr. Lai was the beginning of what I termed the "Reality Campaign." It was a concerted effort by the medical staff to help us, especially me, come to grips with the fact that our daughter was dying. Dr. Smith summed it up best months later in a four-page letter regarding Heidi's hospital stay: "During this time, multiple conversations were held with the parents with regard to the baby's poor prognosis for survival."

Were they wrong? In the physical realm, no. They were thorough, competent medical personnel—some of the best in the country. They were stating obvious facts. Since Chuck did most of the talking in our medical conferences, they knew where he was coming from. He seemed to have a grasp of the situation. Actually, that was his part in the battle plan. God gave him favor with the doctors. He knew what questions to ask. It was he who had the suggestions for the next move most of the time. He was being given the working details for the battle.

I sat quietly in the conferences, hearing the reports, but most of the time not responding emotionally to what they were saying. My part in the battle plan was to focus on what God had said about her. The medical staff did not understand why I was not responding. But it was obvious to them that I was not accepting what they were saying about Heidi. They were mercifully trying to help me accept the medical facts so that I could prepare for her death.

Two hours later, we were back in the same conference room with the neonatologist, Dr. Smith, walking us through the facts regarding Heidi's declining condition.

"Mrs. Watson, I have the impression that you're expecting to walk in here one morning and find everything okay," he explained. I didn't have the nerve to tell him that he was exactly right. I was waiting for my instantaneous miracle. "That's just not going to happen. We all feel like you're not hearing what we're telling you. Mrs. Watson, I need you to repeat back to me what I have told you about Heidi's condition."

"Dr. Smith, I do hear you." It was the most vulnerable I had been in one of our conferences. "What you are saying is that without a miracle my daughter will die. But what I am saying is that I will never give up hope on that miracle as long as there is breath within her."

"It's fine to hope for your miracle, but there has been no indicator that it's going to happen in this case," he gently yet emphatically replied.

Chuck interjected, "Dr. Smith, define the term miracle for me."

"Well, in my practice there have been two babies that have gotten well and left this hospital. I had no explanation why. It was nothing that medical science or I had done. They should have died. There was no medical explanation for their health. That to me is a miracle."

"We're comfortable with that explanation. And Heidi will be your third baby to add to that list," Chuck calmly responded. I sat amazed at his quiet confidence. Just the previous night, we had discussed the difference in our roles. He had confided that it was my word from God on which he was basing his faith. That was difficult, because there had been no direct words for him. Yet he was being given the steps in the plan. I didn't have the slightest clue as to how we were to get from Point A to Point B. I just knew that we were supposed to end up at Point B—miraculously healed baby.

Dr. Smith concluded our meeting, "Well, Mr. Watson, we would all like to see that miracle, but as each day passes, the probability of that becomes less and less." He shook our hands and left the room, still unsure if he had gotten through to us with the facts.

Chuck headed to the waiting room to make a phone call and I headed back to Heidi's bedside. While walking slowly down the hall, the words of a favorite song came to my mind:

> *Rejoice for the steps of a righteous man*
> *They are ordered of God, they are ordered of God.*
> *Rejoice for the steps of a righteous man*
> *They are ordered of God.*
> *In the time of trouble God will uphold him*
> *God will preserve him, God will sustain him*
> *In the time of trouble God will lift him up*
> *So rejoice, your steps are ordered of God.*[3]

It was an upbeat peppy song based on Psalm 37:23. By the time I reached the NICU, my steps had quickened. I was snapping my fingers as I softly sang the song.

Just inside the door of the NICU, I came face to face with Dr. Smith who had entered through another door. I'm sure he had no doubts at that moment. He had obviously not gotten through to this mother. I could imagine his next conversation with Dr. Lai. "Yes, I met with them too. I walked them through all the details of Heidi's condition just like you did.

I even had her repeat back to me what I had told her. Less than two minutes after the conference, she returned to the NICU singing and snapping her fingers. This woman is in 'la-la land.' What do we do to get through to her?"

Two hours later, we were called back to the conference room. Dr. Lai was seated in a chair facing Chuck, Gaylene and me on the soft blue sofa. Gaylene happened to be there visiting and bringing church work for Chuck, so we asked her to meet with us. Three conferences in one day! The Reality Campaign was intense.

He once again summarized her condition, concluding with: "And during the last two hours, it has become evident that the central line we placed for IVs has now infiltrated. This has caused fluid around her lungs. The line has to come out, but the only choice left is to surgically place a catheter in the vein in her neck. Right now if she were to have another cardiac arrest like this afternoon, we would not be able to get emergency medications in her body without an IV line. She is too ill to move to an operating room, so Dr. Ellis will do the surgery at her bedside. There is no indication that she will survive this surgery. But it must be done tonight. This is what I've been trying to explain to you. Problems are mounting by the hour. This is *not* a good situation. I have nothing hopeful to say to you. I'm sorry. You need to sign the approval papers right away so they can get started with the surgery. Any questions?"

"Is there time to see Heidi once again before the surgery?" Chuck tearfully asked.

"Get the papers signed, and the two of you can go in for just a couple of minutes," he replied as he left.

"Vickie, why don't you stay in here with Gaylene while I sign the papers. Then I'll come back for you, and we'll go see Heidi," Chuck suggested.

As he left, I laid my head over on the sofa while Gaylene slipped to the floor beside me. I sobbed. Gaylene put her arms around me. This time there was no peppy song of faith—only pain. "I'm so sorry," Gaylene whispered as we wept together.

Looking back at that moment, it was a picture of a note we had received that week from Bob and Judi, friends through American Airlines. They had quoted a verse from Job 2:13 which now carried tremendous meaning for us. "Then they sat on the ground with him for seven days and seven nights. No one said a word to him, because they saw how great his suffering was." (NIV) The note concluded with, "If you need someone to sit on the ground with you, CALL. We love you. We are praying for you and Heidi Joy." It had touched us deeply.

That's what Gaylene was doing at that moment. Sitting on the ground with me in my grief. Then it hit me. She knew how to hurt with someone because she had experienced pain. It had been two and one-half years since her twenty-six-year-old brother's fatal auto accident. She must have heard similar words about him. Why should she have to witness this? It would be several months later that we would see what God was doing in her life.

"Gaylene, I'm sorry. We weren't thinking about Greg when we asked you to come in here with us. This must be especially hard for you after his death," I reached out to her through my tears.

"It's okay. It really is. I'm just so sorry that you are having to go through this," she wept.

Chuck returned, and the two of us hurried to Heidi's bedside. My swollen, reddened eyes were a signal to the medical staff that their message was finally computing. They were very kind to us as they prepared Heidi for surgery. The surgeon was already with her. He thoroughly explained the procedure before asking us to leave. As we left her bedside, I couldn't help glancing back at her. Would I see her alive again, or was this it?

The next hour was difficult at best. Chuck called home to activate the prayer chain. Dave and Gaylene waited with us.

Several years later, when I read Grandma Boone's journal, I realized how God had also sent people to minister to our parents at the toughest moments.

> Nancy Myers, Nancy Rood and Ken Vaile came over. We ate, cried, prayed, laughed and trusted God for Heidi. Ken went to the store for us and built a fire in the fireplace . . . Pastor Jim came to the house and prayed with us.

The surgery went well. There should be no more problems with veins collapsing. We were able to see her before we left the hospital at midnight. She was sedated and had several new battle scars. Would I ever see my baby without tubes and blood and a fluid-filled body? Would I ever get to dress her in frilly dresses with matching bows in her hair? Would there ever be a full head of hair to hold those bows, rather than large patches of scalp where she had been shaved for IVs? Would I ever see what her face looked like without tape and tubes covering the lower half?

Wednesday, December 4 — Gloria called that morning from Waco and left a message. She would be arriving at noon with a video that we "had to see." This was totally out of character for a woman who planned every step well ahead.

I was emotionally exhausted. The previous day had taken its toll on both of us. My thoughts: *Why would you drive ninety miles to show us a video? It's the last thing I care about at this moment. I don't care how wonderful it may be. We don't have the time or energy for it. I don't want to see your video. Don't you understand? We are living in crisis mode!*

So what did we do when she arrived? She's a female version of Chuck, remember? They're people with a plan. Hard to say "no" to. We gathered in our bedroom to watch the video! I curled up in the blue recliner with my lunch of turkey sandwich and apple slices. Chuck sat on the floor leaning against the arm of the recliner. On our bed were Gloria, Grandma Boone, and Grandma Watson. Lois and her daughter Lori, who had volunteered to answer the phone that day, were seated on the floor.

Within the first ten minutes, I was totally consumed by what Pat Hayes had to say. Lunch sat untouched. The apple turned brown. The bread hardened. But my heart softened as I listened to this mother sharing the battle for her newborn daughter's healing. Her story was akin to what we were experiencing. And we were fighting in similar ways. It was like a report card telling us that we were doing the right things.

Theirs was a long battle with many ups and downs, yet Pat held on to God's word for her child. Her story ended with the audience singing "Emmanuel." It was an anointed moment.

> *Emmanuel, Emmanuel,*
> *His name is called Emmanuel.*
> *God with us, revealed in us!*
> *His name is called Emmanuel.*[4]

There wasn't a dry eye in our bedroom. I closed my eyes and leaned back in the recliner, savoring the moment. Yes, God was with us. I knew it. This was like an oasis in the desert. Tears trickled down my cheeks as I lifted my hands to God in worship, listening to the music and basking in the sweet ministry of the Holy Spirit to my battle-weary, wounded spirit.

The moment was interrupted by Gloria. On her knees at my side, she was tapping on my arm saying, "Open your eyes! You can't miss this part!

I'm sorry to interrupt you, but you have to *see* what's coming next!"

At that moment, a beautiful three-year-old girl with blonde curly hair daintily climbed the steps to the platform to stand beside her mother and join in the singing. She was the picture of life and health. That's what I needed at that moment—a picture. A visual image to hold onto in my mind. God knew I needed it to be a little girl. That was even more powerful.

We were all laughing with joy and crying at the same time. "Isn't she beautiful!"

"Can you believe it? Praise God!"

"That's going to be our Heidi someday!"

Chuck wrapped his arms around me, still laughing and crying. "You're not going to be speaking about hospitality any more, Vickie. You'll be sharing Heidi's story. And she'll walk onto that platform to the glory of God!" I knew he was right. Here was another precious gift from God to carry us through what was happening.

That afternoon as Chuck and I headed to the hospital, I halfway expected to find Heidi healed when we got there. Many times over the past days, I had envisioned walking into the NICU and being greeted by astounded nurses and doctors.

"Mr. and Mrs. Watson," they would say, "the most amazing thing has happened in the last several hours. We don't understand it, but Heidi is fine. Her heart is okay. Her lungs are fully inflated. She's off the respirator and perfectly normal. You can take her home!"

I was expecting a McDonald's® version of a miracle. Drive through . . . fast service . . . instant results. Maybe this would be the day it would happen. Maybe it had even happened while we were watching the video. I had pointed out many "perfect moments" to God for her healing. He seemed to be missing some great opportunities.

But nothing had changed at the hospital when we arrived. In fact, one doctor made the following notation on her chart that day: "Surgical options are limited and prognosis remains guarded." Dr. Lai wrote that it was "also possible tricuspid valve may be too incompetent to ever work adequately. Surgical options all poor."

That night we met Miriam. She was the neighbor of Debbie, who had been in a Bible study group with us the previous year. Debbie and Miriam prayed together often, and their prayers recently had been for Heidi. After several days of this, Miriam sensed that she was to come to the hospital and pray over Heidi.

When she and Debbie arrived, I happened to be in the waiting room visiting with Burtis and Winifred. With both sets of our parents living out of state, we had adopted Burtis and Winifred as our Texas parents for those occasions when we needed a local mom and dad. Burtis had walked through two houses with us several years earlier late one night to help us decide which of the two to buy. We valued their input in our lives.

The previous day's surgical events had left me numb with no more tears. The afternoon video had been a powerful boost to my faith. But my emotional tank was on empty. No more tears. No more reserve for conversations.

I was grateful that this stranger had been praying for my daughter, but yet not in the mood to meet anyone or have to carry on a conversation. My body just wanted to curl up in a corner alone, turn off my brain, and sit. But here was Debbie chatting away about her friend Miriam Watson. No, we weren't related. Yes, it was nice of her to come down. Thanks for your prayers.

Miriam opened a photograph album and began to share the story of her son Michael who was born five and one-half months into her pregnancy. I glanced at a couple of the pictures. He was tiny—fitting in the palm of an adult's hand. As she shared, tears glistened in her eyes. Debbie began to weep and patted my knee throughout the story.

My inward response? *Stop weeping, Debbie, and stop patting my knee. It's driving me crazy. I don't have any tears left, and I don't want to listen to someone else crying for me.*

My mind drifted from Miriam's words to her face. You know how we women are at analyzing each other. She was beautiful. Although petite in size, heads would turn if she walked into a room. There was nothing petite about her hair, her eyes, or her nails. Her long thick head of hair was teased adding quite a few inches to her height. Her large eyes seemed even bigger with the dramatic make-up. And her brightly colored fingernails could have been weapons. Her smooth Costa Rican skin was flawless. Bright earrings matched the hot pink in her outfit. She spoke with intensity, and the word "Watson" snapped my focus back to what she was saying.

"I have three Watson boys and had also wanted a girl. Yesterday afternoon as I was praying for Heidi, the Lord said to me, 'This is the Watson baby girl that you have prayed for. You are to intercede for her as if she were your own.' So that's why I'm here."

Those words certainly caught my attention. *God, what am I supposed to do? I'm too tired to figure this one out. Did you send Miriam here, or is this a distraction? Help!*

At that moment Chuck came out to see why I had not returned. I introduced them and explained that Miriam had come to pray for Heidi. Chuck sensed my hesitation and smoothly handled the situation. "Vickie, why don't you go on in and be with Heidi, so she won't be alone. Burtis, Winifred, and I will visit with Miriam and Debbie."

Thank you, God. I knew Chuck would not send her back to Heidi's bedside, unless he sensed that it was right. He was also fishing for Burtis' and Winifred's input in the matter. As I walked down the hallway I relaxed, thankful for Chuck's discerning spirit about people.

She certainly doesn't look like God's messenger to me! With that thought, the Holy Spirit quietly said to me, "Who are you to say what my messenger will look like? You're in a pretty desperate situation right now."

Oooh! Message received. I certainly wasn't in a place to be choosy. *God, if she's from you, send her on back to the NICU.*

Ten minutes later, Chuck brought Miriam back and showed her how to scrub in and gown. Only two people were allowed at her bedside unless one was a minister. So Chuck brought her back to pray and then left. She immediately walked to Heidi's side, not intimidated at all by the machinery and tubes. It was obvious that she had spent long days in the NICU with her own baby. Laying her hand on Heidi's chest, she began to pray. Any doubts I had were gone within seconds. The gentleness of her conversation was gone, and there was a profound authority in her praying. I had never heard anyone pray that forcefully. She told Satan where he could go, since he was finished with his assignment on this baby. She claimed God's word and His healing power for Heidi. She commissioned warrior angels and ministering angels to be at her side to carry out God's work. I felt the power—the electricity—in the air. This woman knew God intimately and understood how to fight spiritual battles. She didn't waste time. Neither was she timid. She was there for about thirty minutes. I watched with grateful astonishment.

Chuck came back to join us just as Miriam finished praying. She looked up at both of us with tears streaming down her cheeks and eyes glowing. I'll never forget her emphatic words. "Thus saith the Lord, 'She shall live and shall not die. I have not sent my death angel unto her. But I have created her for life. **She shall live!**'"

With tears streaming down our faces, we held on to her every word. Miriam Watson was a prophet sent from God with His message for us.

"There's one other thing I sense that I'm to tell you. God has said that she will live, but she may get worse before she gets better. In fact, that is what will happen, but you are not to fear. God is in control. She shall live and not die!"

I thought Chuck was going to shake her when she said the part about getting worse before she got better. It didn't seem possible for her to be any worse and still be alive. Maybe that part of the prophecy wouldn't happen. But the bottom line was that God had said she would live.

As we hugged good-bye, she promised to continue in prayer for Heidi. She and her family were leaving in two days to spend a month in Costa Rica for the holidays. She would be back to see Heidi as soon as they returned in January.

Chuck walked her back to the waiting room. I sat in stunned silence. A prophet! God had sent a prophet with the same last name as ours to Heidi's bedside. And the packaging! He had certainly changed His packaging since Isaiah and Jeremiah. But I wasn't complaining. Just very grateful for another confirmation of His Word for Heidi.

When Chuck returned, he got a good laugh when I shared what the Holy Spirit said about what His messenger would look like. What a sense of humor God has!

"I wish she wasn't leaving the country for a month," Chuck said. "That part about things getting worse before they get better—if that's true, I want her here praying when that happens. But I hope it doesn't happen. I don't see how she could get any worse."

"Chuck, I don't think God is going to let us depend on anything or anyone except Him. He has made it clear that He will not share His glory with another. Maybe that's why she's out of the picture for now. But I'm like you. I still wish she was going to be here for at least another week."

Thursday, December 5 — That afternoon at the hospital, I decided it was time to add more to Heidi's tape from me. Leaving her in her Daddy's care, I went to my favorite quiet spot—the chapel. I sang songs—"Jesus

Loves Me," "Oh How He Loves You and Me," "God is the Strength of My Heart," "Praise the Name of Jesus," and many others. Then I added the Mommy part. The idea had come after watching the video on Wednesday. The words spilled from my heart:

> Know in your spirit, Heidi, that He is Jehovah. He is your provider. He is your healer. Know that the Lord God, it is He that delivers you. He is your comforter, Heidi. You rest in His arms. Rest in the arms of Jesus.
>
> He is the one who has created within you a new heart. He is the one who has softened your lungs and has breathed life into those lungs. Life and health and healing and wholeness. And He is the One who has raised you up, so that you will walk out of here with us, in our arms, healthy, whole, with a perfect heart in every way for the glory of God. Know that in your spirit.
>
> And, Heidi, I look forward to the days ahead with you. There are the cutest little black patent leather shoes at home and the dresses. And we're going to do hair bows. We're going to wash your hair and let it form into those beautiful curls and ringlets that God gave to you. We're going to go for walks around the neighborhood. Sterling and I will pull you in the red wagon.
>
> When Daddy gets home from work, we'll all get on the bicycle built for two. You'll be strapped in the snuggle carrier on Daddy's chest, and Sterling will be in the child seat behind me. We'll go for rides around the neighborhood, and we'll show you God's creation. We'll show you the birds and the sky and the flowers and the beauty in what He has created.
>
> There are seventy-two yellow pansies smiling and wait-

ing for you to come home. Your flag is flying from the flag-pole. It says, "Happy Birthday, Heidi," and it will continue to fly until you come home. Until we bring you into the house where your cradle is ready for you. You'll sleep there. The diapers are ready. Everything is ready. Ohhh, we long for that day. And we're looking forward to it. Heidi, it is coming because of what Jesus has done. What He has done in your life and continues to do. You are healed, honey. You are whole by the blood of the lamb of Jesus.

You'll go to the ranch with us and see the cows and horses. When we go to Ohio, Uncle Don will take us for rides in the wagon. You'll see the farm where your Daddy grew up. When we go to Mississippi, you'll swing in the backyard. Grandpa will put you in the little wagon behind his riding lawn mower and pull you around the yard. You'll giggle and laugh. We'll go to family reunions at the beach, and you'll stick your toes in the sand. We'll take your diaper off, and you'll sit in the sand on your little bottom. We'll build sand castles. And the waves will come up and tickle your toes. And all those aunts and uncles will hug you and kiss on you. They'll probably bounce you around. You'll meet more relatives than you ever knew you could have.

We look forward to those days, Heidi. And I see you—I see the day, honey, when we will share what God has done for you. God will open the doors. And I won't be talking about hospitality any more, but about what God has done in our family's life. And when we get through sharing, Daddy will bring you and Sterling up those steps, and we'll stand there and praise God. You'll clap your hands in praise to God and lift your hands in praise to Him. And we'll sing to the praise and glory of God for what He has done, Heidi. For what He has done in every member of our family through His power. The miracle of Heidi.

Miracle Heidi. Your Daddy said today that that's going to be your nickname. And it fits . . . Heidi, we love you SO much. We look forward to the years ahead with you that God gives to us. We love you, honey. Heidi Joy Watson— battle maiden of delight. You are a blessing, honey.

Returning to her bedside an hour later, I inserted the freshly recorded cassette into the player at Heidi's bedside. "Guess what, Heidi, more good news. Just listen to what's ahead for you. It's going to be fun!" It was as much of a boost for me as for her.

Meanwhile, the Reality Campaign continued. Now they were working on the grandparents. Grandma Boone's journal recorded:

They turned Heidi on her stomach for the first time. Bile fluid (green) poured into her tube . . . valium . . . Our nurse came over and talked to me about Heidi and her future.

That night Mother called my brother Dan in Bourbonnais, Illinois. He pastors the College Church at Olivet Nazarene University where Chuck had graduated. The church had been a faithful part of Heidi's prayer support team, and Mother kept them updated. After her conversation with the nurse about Heidi's future, Mother asked Dan to call or write a letter to help me face the possibility that Heidi might not make it. A year later, Dan confessed to me that he had written the letter, but could not bring himself to mail it. We were all glad that he hadn't.

Friday, December 6 — The "walk of faith" was a yo-yo experience for all of us. Up and down. Up and down. Dr. Smith called our home that morning with more bad news. Mother's journal recorded it:

> Doctors called and said they suspect Heidi may have brain damage. They will do cat scan and EEG tonight and in the morning. They have done all they can do. Unless God performs a miracle, she can't make it. We expect a Miracle.

That morning Adrienne brought a gift for Heidi by the house. It was a green corduroy jumper with red trim and a white blouse—very German, just like Heidi's name. Size four toddler. She had bought a larger size as a symbol of her faith. The attached card read, "Yes, Vickie, I *do* believe that Heidi will make it—will be healed—and will keep you busy chasing after her when she wears this dress. It looks like it was especially made for her. With my love and my faith joining yours, Adrienne."

Meanwhile, the Reality Campaign continued. It was played out in many arenas, intensified by the fact that Heidi did not open her eyes or respond in any way for three days following the surgery.

That afternoon as Heidi lay motionless, her nurse Katie* initiated a conversation with me.

"Mrs. Watson, how do you think Heidi is doing medically?"

"I understand that she is in serious condition," I mumbled, immediately aware that I wanted to end the interchange as quickly as possible.

"Well, would you say that she is the same or better or worse?" she pressed.

"I am fully aware of what her condition is," I repeated wearily.

"How would you describe her condition?" she pressed further.

---

* fictitious name.

"Katie, I understand what you're saying and what you're trying to make me say. Yes, short of a miracle, my daughter will not live. But I know what God told me about her before she was ever born. I will never give up hope as long as there is breath within her. Never!" I responded emphatically.

"Mrs. Watson, we are aware that this is a stressful time for you and your husband. It puts tremendous stress on any marriage. The divorce rate of NICU parents is extremely high. You may need to seek help during these days. How is your marriage holding up?"

"Our marriage has never known such strength and oneness as we are experiencing through this crisis," I proudly reported. "My marriage is fine, thank you."

We were interrupted by the voice over the intercom announcing that all visitors should leave during the nurses' change of shift. I walked out sobbing, grateful for the interruption, and sought out Chuck's shoulder in the waiting room.

Although our marriage had always been good, it was true. I had never sensed such a oneness—operating like one well-oiled, finely tuned piece of machinery. We were two parts, each having different functions, but we made up a complete unit. Chuck had the battle plan, and I had the faith. The hospital days were a confirmation of the strength of our marriage. The stress in that area would come much later.

There was also another conference with Dr. Smith that afternoon. My journal reflected the tone of the meeting:

> **Dr. Smith's report:** Muscle tone and activity not good; not as good as one week ago; doing EEG and head sonogram to test for brain damage.
>
> **God's report:** (silence)
>
> **Dr. Smith's report:** We can't get her any lower than 20

beats per minute on respirator.

GOD'S *report:* *(silence)*

Dr. Smith's *report:* Lungs not as good today as yesterday; sees different part of right lung collapse each day; won't resolve until right atrium of heart goes down, if it ever does; not much more we can do to keep lung expanded except continue breathing treatments.

GOD'S *report:* *(silence)*

Dr. Smith's *report:* Problems are now mounting up —
- can't digest feedings
- infection in blood
- poor muscle tone—brain damage?
- anything we do to try to relieve one problem causes another.

GOD'S *report:* *(silence)*

Dr. Smith's *report:* We're less optimistic with each day; how much have you thought about her dying?

GOD'S *report:* *(silence)*

Dr. Smith's *report:* It's fine to hang on to your miracle, but you've got to prepare yourself for the other possibility.

GOD'S *report:* *(silence)*

Dr. Smith's *report:* As time goes on, we are less and less hopeful that she will go home.

GOD'S *report:* *(silence)*

Dr. Smith's *report:* I wish I had something good to tell you, but I don't.

The "God" spaces on the page were empty. I had nothing to write there. In fact, I didn't journal again for eleven months. It was difficult enough to make it through each day. I could no longer re-live the events to journal them. It was far too painful.

How much have you thought about her dying?

I Will Not! I was hanging on. But the rope was getting threadbare. And my arms were losing strength.

Chapter Eight

How Do You Want Her To Die?

Saturday, December 7 — Finally some good news! The tests showed no signs of brain damage! Heidi opened her eyes for the first time since Tuesday. The final conclusion was that her body had probably not been able to handle the sedation during and following the surgery.

Dr. Lai's written notes regarding that day:

> Heidi on intubated ventilation and prostaglandin infusion. Overall status remains guarded . . . Had further discussions with parents. Emphasized that Heidi may not survive neonatal period unless there is significant change in present status. Surgery is less of realistic option after discussions with surgeons in Dallas and Houston.

That afternoon Pat Pittman walked into our lives. She had worked on a computer project with our mutual friend Pam, who had shared Heidi's story with her. Pat's ministry was intercession—especially for babies. Pam had told us that Pat would come to the hospital Friday night, so I had been a little disappointed when Pat had called to say that she wouldn't be there that night. The reason: "I feel that I'm to pray and fast for twenty-four hours before I come." She took her gifting from the Lord seriously. I couldn't complain about anyone who wanted to pray and fast for my child before coming to lay hands on her in prayer.

So I was glad to finally meet her in person when she and her husband

Mike arrived early Saturday evening. Tall, thin, long black hair, intense dark eyes. She was a mixture of shyness (that's why she liked praying for babies) and boldness in the things of the Lord. Her down-to-earth sense of humor was a surprising contrast to the intensity of her prayer life. When God called her to intercede for a baby, she knew that would mean hours of prayer daily and sleepless nights spent travailing in prayer. Committing to pray for Heidi and walk this journey with us—total strangers—was a sacrifice of love.

The four of us talked in the waiting room for awhile, getting acquainted and sharing more of Heidi's history. Very few visitors were allowed in the NICU—then only one at a time with one of the parents. Pat and I went in to Heidi's bedside. She spent about an hour in prayer with Heidi that evening as I sat in the rocker nearby. I sensed the presence and power of the Lord, although I never heard her words. It didn't matter. We didn't even talk that much as she left that night. But I vividly remember her parting words, "God says that she will live. She will not die."

Over the following days, each time we talked to Pat by telephone, she recorded the conversations on her answering machine tape, filling ten tapes over a seven week period. Three years later on my fortieth birthday, she gave me a three ring binder bearing a picture of a precious lamb. The binder contained one hundred eighty-two typed pages of the transcripts of those phone conversations. It is among my most valued possessions. As I wrote this book, I understood how God had paved the way back in the midst of the battle.

Sunday, December 8 — Pat called our home around noon to see about Heidi, so I hooked up a three-way phone conversation with my sister Rose Annette who was at the hospital. Heidi had rested comfortably most of the morning. For the first time, she had been able to maintain on a respirator rate of 15 for more than an hour.

"I feel good about her today," reported Rose Annette. "I didn't even see her eyes Friday. They didn't open at all that day. There was not a lot of movement. And she definitely has had movement today. She's tried to lift her head. Dad walked off at one point, and it was like 'Where are you going?' She followed him. She got her head up a little, but she couldn't get it turned."

Pat: "Is she still trying to move her arms and legs?"

Rose Annette: "She is moving arms and legs."

Pat: "What are they going to do about that? She'll be trying to get that tube out of her mouth."

Rose Annette: "I've watched that this morning, because her little arms are moving very much, and her little legs are kicking. She definitely shows some signs of a normal little girl."

Vickie: "That will be interesting to see. They may have to pin her hands down. If we're sitting there, they allow us to hold her hands and watch her with it. She likes holding your hand. So that's fine. But during the one-hour nursing shift change each morning and evening, I'm not sure what they'll do. I heard one of the therapists say that if she got a hold of it, she's strong enough now to pull out the respirator tube."

Pat: "She may not need that tube much longer."

Vickie: "Yes, if they're coming down that fast on the respirator rate, as long as they're getting good blood gases. Rose Annette, last night Chuck said that they got the best blood gas they've ever gotten . . . They look at the blood gas level to bring the respirator down. So hitting 15 on the respirator is significant. If the blood gas continues to be good, they would bring it down to 10, then to 5. They said if we hit 5 on the respirator and she's stable, we're ready to turn off the respirator."

Rose Annette: "Oh, really good. That's what I'm ready for."

Vickie and Pat: "Yeah!!!"

Rose Annette: "She's had church this morning. We had soft worship and then praise. Mommy was her preacher. We listened to your tape. We did what we thought they would be doing at church. Then we had scripture and prayer, so we got it all in this morning."

Vickie: "Good, Sis! . . ."

Rose Annette: "Dr. Smith was in earlier and asked about Chuck and you. He said that he would talk to you this afternoon . . . Dr. Lai came in, and Dad asked how his grand-daughter was doing. He said, 'She's no better. She's definitely not any worse. You know at this point, we're just trying to strengthen her. We do feel like she'll do that.' . . . He was not negative. I was surprised."

Vickie: "He's changed . . . I mean, he's the one who said, 'You have *got* to hear what we're saying.' And he was incredibly blunt. Gaylene was there at the time. We wanted someone else with us, because our emotions that night were so raw. Yesterday I talked to somebody who had talked to her. Gaylene said that it was 'awful . . . the most awful stuff I've ever heard.' Then when we met with Dr. Lai last night, he was saying, 'We don't see any improvement, but I haven't given up hope.' And I thought, 'This is Dr. Lai?' . . ."

Rose Annette: "Dr. Smith is the same way . . . Friday night he said, 'We definitely have not given up hope on her by any means.'. . ."

Pat: "Yesterday before I left to come to the hospital, I was praying, and the Lord said, 'When the doctors get to the point they've done all they can do, then stand back and watch My glory fall.' And I said, 'Okay, we'll watch.' Then when I was getting ready to leave, He said that in the next twenty-four hours, they will see some major changes. And they will have to know that it's the Lord. We're two hours away now from twenty-four hours, and a lot has happened in twenty-four hours."

Vickie: "Yes. She's come from 30 to 15 on the respirator. Especially the 15 is significant. The doctor kept saying 'We can't get her down to 15 without her going into distress. I can't just cut her. I mean we could, but it would be foolish to just say that we had gotten her to 20 on the respirator, so let's try her without it. That's like telling a person with a broken leg to go run the fifty-yard dash. You've got to go in increments.' . . ."

Pat: "What's the deal with the valium . . . morphine? . . ."

Vickie: "Chuck just reminded me . . . The nurses have told him that any time an adult or child is on a respirator, they will normally keep them on some kind of sedative just to help them manage that tube. Otherwise, it's so hard for them to handle the tube being down their throat . . ."

Pat: ". . . Last night when I laid down, I asked the Lord if there was anything I needed to do to follow up. And the one thing He said to me was that Satan could come against her again symptomatically. It would not be a real attack. You would see symptoms that would appear that something is going on. He said to warn you that if you see the appearance of evil, the appearance of an attack, to rebuke the symptoms, because Satan has no more ground in her. So it would be purely a symptom. Rebuke the symptom, because the nurses and doctors are going to react to what symptoms they see in her. They're not going to know the difference, but you will . . . Rose, when you're in there and she starts to go into distress, and you feel like she's in any kind of pain at all, particularly if you see her stomach kind of quiver—like yesterday her stomach would almost vibrate—if you see that, put your hand on her stomach and rebuke the demon of pain. Rebuke it out of her in Jesus' name, and she'll stop. She did that two or three times yesterday, and I did that, and she stopped instantly. So Satan is putting symptoms on her, I think, so that the attendants will respond and do things that she doesn't need done to her. If you rebuke the symptoms he has no more ground there."

Rose Annette: "Yes, I feel that very strongly. He's through."

Pat: "She's protected. She's in the hands of God. And anything you see like that, just get your hands on her and rebuke whatever demon is coming against her. Then that symptom will cease, and they won't have to do anything else. And you can even speak peace into her where that tube is concerned. Just get down in her face and command her to open her eyes and look at you in Jesus' name. Speak into her spirit. Tell her to receive that tube and leave it alone, to let it stay there until the Lord takes it out, not to fight it. And when the Lord's ready to take it out, He'll have it removed. But if she fights it, they're going to see that as something else. So she needs to fight off the infection. She needs to fight off infirmity. But she doesn't need to fight the treatment, because the more calm she is about that, the quicker they're going to take it out. She won't understand that in the natural, but you speak to her spirit. She will understand that . . . Ask the Holy Spirit to give her peace so she won't fight that tube."

As I drove to the hospital an hour later, there was another piece of good news. It was a sunshiny, crisp Sunday afternoon. Chuck was spending some time with Sterling and would be riding down later with friends. So it was one of the rare times that I went alone.

My mind was on Sterling as I drove along Bedford-Euless Road about a mile from home. How was this affecting him? He seemed secure and content. He was enjoying the time with his three grandparents. I just didn't want to forget him in the midst of the Heidi crisis. Several people had told me at church that morning that they were praying for Sterling. God certainly seemed to be covering all bases.

As I passed the Bedford Boys' Ranch, something caught my eye. They had changed their marquee advertising an upcoming play. We had memorized every detail of the drive to the hospital over the past weeks. So any minute change was obvious to us on our daily trek. The brick sign was perched on a grassy knoll, nestled among the trees. The message of its black letters caused me to take a second look: "On Stage—Heidi, December 14-22."

I slowed down to be sure. Yes, the sign read "On Stage—Heidi, December 14-22." But the honking of horns forced me to keep moving. *God, is this from you? Am I pulling things out of the air? Or are you using billboards these days? Is this a coincidence?*

I knew within seconds. It was from Him! It was as if He were sitting in the van with me, arm around my shoulder and pointing to the sign. "Just wanted you to know what's ahead," He reassured me.

My mind went into fast forward. He had given me a message and I knew what to do with it. No need for explanation. I knew exactly what this meant. For the past two Sunday mornings, I had heard the announcement in church: "Baby dedication on Sunday morning, December 22." Each time I had sat there wondering. *Do I dare dream that Heidi will be a part of that dedication? She will be a month old by then. God has said that her life will be a miracle. Surely it will be done by then. Can that be our date to hope for? It seems like a long ways off right now, but if I just knew that the end of this ordeal were in sight.*

Here was my answer. What else could "On Stage—Heidi, December 14-22" mean? And the dates fit perfectly. She would be healed and come home from the hospital sometime during the week following the fourteenth. That was only six days away. The culmination would be her dedication on December 22. What a Christmas this would be! Finally, the end was in sight!

When I arrived at the hospital, she looked great. But over the next hours, a couple of things began to concern me. I left the following message on Pat's answering machine at 5:36 p.m.:

"Pat, this is Vickie. Heidi seems to be doing much better this afternoon. The one thing I have not been able to do is to get her eyes open to come against the symptoms. Right at this point, her blood gas is much worse. Her heart rate is slowing down, so they took extra blood gas levels to check that. I still feel like it's symptoms, but I was only able to get her to open one eye just a slit, and I didn't like the look I saw. But I couldn't get her to keep it open. We're still down to 15 on the rate, but they're saying we may have to go back up because of the heart slowing down a little. There's a chance her heart may be resting . . . Just wanted to give you an update, okay. Bye."

Her husband Mike picked up the phone at the end of my message, and we talked briefly. When Pat returned the call an hour later, a few more pieces of the puzzle started fitting as we talked:

Vickie: " . . . There was one other thing I told Mike. This may not mean anything at all. But one thing I see—in my spirit, I think—across her forehead, there's a duskiness. That's the only word I know to describe it. Her coloring looks great from there down, but across her forehead this afternoon, I've seen a duskiness."

Pat: "Well, he told me that, and I immediately came in here and started praying. It does mean something . . . I hear two things in my spirit. First of all, when we talked last night, you told me about a recurring dream you had during pregnancy—about your baby dying. Did you have a fear that she was going to die?"

Vickie: "Oh, yes."

Pat: "Has anyone prayed over you and broken that curse off of you?"

Vickie: "No, I never told anyone."

Pat: "Okay. Then what's happening is called transference of spirits. Are you familiar with that?"

Vickie: "Yes, I think I know what you mean. They're within me and coming to her?"

Pat: "Yes. And when you had those dreams, that curse entered the womb through you. So that curse of death that we prayed off of her last night is still attached to you. You need to be delivered from that."

Vickie: "Okay."

Pat: "Because what's happening is when you go in and touch her, that

spirit—that little demon—is jumping off onto her. That spirit is transfer-
ring because she was doing so well this afternoon. The morphine—yeah,
that could keep her from opening her eyes. But just the fact that in your
spirit, you can tell something is wrong. And the grayness across the forehead, to me, says that something has attached. The only way it can
attach—Satan cannot send anything to her, because she's covered by the
Blood. She's loosed from Satan. But she can receive a transference of spirits from somebody touching her that has a spirit on her. That's the reason
that anybody in a prayer ministry at all will tell you to be very careful
who you let lay hands on you. If that person is not clean themselves, they
can transfer spirits onto you. So, don't let just anybody pray over you. If
you don't know that they're clean, don't let them touch you . . ."

We then made logistical plans for Mike and Pat to come to the hospital and pray later that night. Our conversation ended with—

Pat: ". . . Satan has a foothold there that has to be broken off again.
Once that's bound off, she will start improving again. I see this totally at
this point now as a spiritual battle. You know, it was physical to start
with. There were obviously physical problems, and only the Lord knows
why the problems came. That's not our business. All we know is what to
do after we get here. So, that's the only thing that the Lord told me—if
that had never been broken off of you, that needs to be dealt with . . .
Well, we'll be up there about eight o'clock."

Our prayer time late that night in the hospital chapel was powerful.
The fear of Heidi dying was gone. Those pregnancy dreams no longer
held any power over me. We were moving in the right direction. And
God was changing me in the process.

I returned to Heidi's room with a new boldness. It was day eighteen
of her life. Approaching her bedside, I addressed Mary our nurse for the
night. "You know, I'd really like to hold her tonight. I've just held her the

one time."

As Heidi snuggled down into my arms, she showed her approval by an improved heart rate and oxygen saturation levels. Chuck and Mary beamed. Forty-five minutes later, I reluctantly placed her back in bed, and we said good night. Leaving her there each night was so difficult. It ran against the grain of every mothering instinct within me.

Thirty minutes later as we tiptoed through our kitchen into the front entryway leading to our bedroom, we were welcomed by a beautiful sight. The twinkling white lights on our eight-foot Christmas tree beckoned us into the living room. It was decked with the usual angels, lace-trimmed bows, and beaded hearts. Our parents and care group members had spent the evening decorating the house for Christmas.

Annie, a lady from church who cleaned houses, had also showed up. Mother's journal described her as an "angel. She cleaned the house, changed beds and did everything—laundry, dishes, vacuuming and all." A note from Annie greeted us:

> I will finish cleaning and doing laundry when I come back tomorrow afternoon at one o'clock . . . Thanks for letting me come over and help you. It's something I *needed* to do. Let me encourage you to continue to be *strong*. People are watching you, and you are setting a good example for others. You never know who you might touch. You and your precious daughter *matter* more than we know. You have encouraged me, and I'm blessed to know you! Love much, Annie

Thanks for *letting* me clean your house? Here was another nugget about ministry. Annie was operating within her gifting and under the Holy Spirit's direction. It was a natural thing to her, or rather a supernatural thing. She had been a blessing to our household that evening. And who was ministered to? Both giver and receiver.

We had learned much about ministry in the past years by being on the giving end. But we were now learning far more from the receiving end.

Monday, December 9 — Mother's report of the previous night let us know that the roller coaster ride was not over yet. Her journal showed what had happened as we slept:

> Heidi is not doing well. They had to pull the breathing tube out and suction. Heart rate went to 102. At 12:48 a.m. her heart rate is 111. Mary is her nurse tonight . . . Respirator is on 30 and oxygen at 21%. The respirator went down to 15 today, but they had to push it back up because of bad blood gases.

The doctor's notes on her chart reflected the same:

> Day 19 of age with essentially no signs of improvement in cardiopulmonary status. Remains ventilator dependent . . . Requires PGE [prostaglandin] to maintain open PDA [heart duct] for pulmonary flow and acceptable saturations. Medical management obviously is not helping. Discussed options (surgically) with cardiology who will pursue them and talk to parents. Prognosis remains very poor.

Meanwhile Pat's answering machine recorded the following prophecy around noon during a prayer time between Pat and her prayer partner Carol:

Carol: "*She shall be an example of My Praise . . . Thou shalt live and thou shalt not die! I have not loosed my death angels on this baby! Hallelujah . . . Sing forth praises out of your mouth . . . This baby was saved before she even entered the womb, and she's sure saved coming out of the womb. She shall live and she shall not die!!! I have a work to be done in her and for her and by My Spirit for the elders of the Church to stand by and see this miracle. Thank you, Father. Thank you, Jesus . . . Lord, we praise you. This is truly a miracle.*"

At the end of their prayer, Carol suggested that our pastoral staff anoint and pray over a prayer cloth or baby pillow to be placed on Heidi's torso. It was to be a covering representing the total shelter of the Lord's hand.

An hour later, Carol called Pat once again.

Carol: "I called to tell you what else the Lord told me about our baby girl. What is that baby's name?"

Pat: "Heidi Joy. The name Heidi means 'Battle Maiden.'"

Carol: "Oh, let me tell you—I did not know that. When I get through telling you what the Lord told me about this baby . . . *[He says we're talking about] binding and loosing. Command evil spirits to be gone. Then loose the powers of prayer to work. That shakes the powers of darkness, hell, and destruction. They have to be loosed themselves, because My Word says so. They have attached themselves to the heart of My little baby girl, and (get this) wrongfully so. But now that you've prayed the prayer of agreement and the prayer of faith, they had to go and she's fine now. All that worry over nothing. Didn't I tell you My Word works? For if it's in the Bible, then I told you so. She shall live and not die. Prayers will not be in vain. She shall be wise and joyful. Peace, My peace I give unto her. Blessings upon blessings, she shall receive. Amen.* So that's what He told me. He kept calling her Joy, and

I didn't know that [was part of her name]."

Early that evening, I sat on the floor in the waiting room at a pay phone listening to the taped prayer as Pat played it for me. Then Chuck and I switched places, and he listened while I returned to Heidi's bedside. The prayer cloth. The words of prophecy. These were not everyday occurrences in our lives. But were we open? Yes. When you're fighting for your baby's life, you become open to any avenue God may choose to use. It doesn't have to fall within your self-imposed "spiritual comfort zone." It just has to be from God.

What I was hearing in that prophecy was once again in sharp contrast to what Dr. Smith had told us in our conference that afternoon. There we were again on the blue sofa in the conference room facing him as he pulled his chair closer. I don't think I'll ever want to own a blue sofa! Talk about difficult memories!

"I need to summarize for you where we are," he began. "We have basically come down to a decision-making point. You need to decide how you want your daughter to die. Her medical team concurs that she will not live, but you do have some choices about how she will die."

Was I hearing him right? Nothing in life prepares you to make a decision like that. You never dream that you will be asked to do it! *How do I want my child to die?* I couldn't believe we were hearing these words. Yet he was speaking reality in the natural realm. That's the way things were. And he was trying to help us deal with the facts.

"There are three choices," he continued. "Option one: If you choose to do nothing, waiting for improvement, she will probably die from a secondary cause such as infection or other complications. We see that happen many times. With her weakened condition, she couldn't fight off much. Option two: You have talked with various heart surgeons across the nation. Dr. Leonard in Dallas has discussed with you the possibility of a radical heart surgery in which the structure of the heart is changed. He is willing to do that, although he has made it clear that no child has ever survived the surgery. This would be a last-ditch effort on your part, but we would certainly understand if you wanted to try it. Option three: We could send her to Dallas for a possible heart transplant. If Heidi should survive until a donor heart were found, she would not survive the transplant surgery. But again, we would understand if you needed to try this route, just to know that you had tried everything possible.

"But we must have a decision from you. Time is running out. With the way things have been going, options two and three could cease to be alternatives if she gets any worse. You must decide. How do you want her to die?" The medical team had been leading us to this point over the past week. And now it was here. There was no more buying of time. It was clear that he wanted a decision now.

"Vickie and I would like to discuss this and let you know in an hour," Chuck responded, obviously frustrated.

"That will be fine. But we must have some definitive decision this afternoon. We can't wait any longer," he replied as he left.

Over the next hour we talked much, cried much, and prayed much. We both felt backed into a corner and abandoned. Like time was running out, and we had been left without any viable options.

God, where are you? Don't you know we have to give them an answer in an hour? This is the eleventh hour and we aren't hearing from you.

"The only thing I feel is that we're to wait," I hesitantly admitted to Chuck. "I can't even tell you what I'm basing that on. But I just keep thinking that we're to give it thirty days. I don't know why. I don't even know if it's right. But it's the only thing I have to go on right now. I wish God would give us some kind of sign, some kind of confirmation. The stakes are too high to risk making a wrong decision. This is our child's life we're talking about!"

In the waiting room we talked with Pastor Jim, Pastor Travis, Dave, Mike, and Kaylene. As we discussed it, someone suggested that each person share what he would do if it were his child. Pastor Travis wisely responded, "That's helpful in many decisions in life. But suppose what I would do for my child is wrong for Heidi? This is far too important. No, we have to know what God desires for Heidi's situation—how *He* wants to handle this."

As they continued talking, I flipped through my Bible looking at Scriptures I had underlined over the past three weeks. *God, please confirm something to us through Your Word. We have to hear from you. My feeling that we should wait thirty days isn't enough to go on.*

Then I found it. Or rather, He showed it to me. His confirmation was in Hebrews 4:12-16:

> For the word of God is living and active and sharper than any two-edged sword, and piercing as far as the division of soul and spirit, of both joints and marrow, and able to judge the thoughts and intentions of the heart. And there is no creature hidden from His sight, but all things are open and laid bare to the eyes of Him with whom we have to do. Since then we have a great high priest who has passed through the heavens, Jesus the Son of God, let us hold fast our confession. For we do not have a high priest who cannot sympathize with our weaknesses, but one who has been tempted in all things as we are, yet without sin. Let us therefore draw near with confidence to the throne of grace, that we may receive mercy and may find grace to help in time of need. (NASB)

"Chuck, look at this. Here it is!" I exclaimed, reading the verses aloud to them. "Verse 12 says that 'the word of God is living and active and sharper than any two-edged sword.' That's the knife of surgery! Are we against surgery? No. God works through a surgeon's skillful hands many times. But what is He saying about surgery for *this* situation? No. He will not share His glory with another. He is going to do it in such a way that all will undeniably know it was His hand that healed Heidi. His word is sharper than the sword of surgery for this circumstance. No surgery!"

How do you want her to die? We chose to wait for God's intervention.

There were two other encouraging moments that day. Earlier that afternoon Chuck and I had discussed holding Heidi. "You know, I've been wondering if we should just say, 'Could we hold her once a day when you pick her up to weigh her?'"

"I've been thinking the same thing," he responded. This wasn't unusual. We were a unit trekking together. "We need to be holding her more. She needs our touch."

When he approached Nurse Sarah with the idea, she liked it. "Well, you know, we were talking about that. I don't see why not. But no one except the parents. And only as long as she handles it well. Let's try it for five minutes."

As Chuck motioned me to the wooden rocker by her bedside, I shook my head. "No, it's your turn. I've held her twice. You've waited long enough." As Heidi was placed in his arms for the first time, we both wept. Heidi snuggled. And once again her breathing and heart rate improved. He held her for an hour that night as she slept peacefully. Then I held her for forty-five minutes. The only time she got upset was when we placed her back on her bed.

Later that evening in the waiting room one of the other "NICU dads" approached Chuck hesitantly. His child's bed was near Heidi's, separated only by a cabinet holding her medical supplies and machinery.

"I uh—I want to tell you something. And I hope you won't be offended. We are Christians and I have sensed that you are a man of God," he began.

"Well, you're right that we're Christians. And we're open to anything God wants to tell us," Chuck replied.

"We were praying for our baby earlier tonight with another couple. During the prayer time, we felt that we were to be praying for your daughter also. As soon as we started praying for her, the Holy Spirit told me, 'God has a calling on that baby. He has something special for her.' So I just wanted to share that as a word of encouragement."

"Well, it fits right in line with everything else God has been showing us," Chuck responded enthusiastically.

The report card? *Spiritually:* The message was coming through loud and clear. She shall live! *Medically:* There was no lasting sign of improvement. Nothing to give us any hope.

Tuesday, December 10 — Grandpa Boone and substitute "Grandpa Ed" started their hospital shift at 7:00 that morning. Grandpa Ed was becoming a regular at the hospital. Every Sunday at church you saw him with a toddler in his arms or chasing after him. He loved toddlers. But by his own admission, babies were not his thing. His explanation: "I don't like to fool with them until they can talk and run around. I like them even better if they're house broken." After staying with Dad at the hospital a couple of Saturdays, Ed started showing up more and more. He would join Dad many times in the middle of the day with the explanation, "I was in the area and really didn't have any more sales calls that *had* to be made today." Or, "sales have been so good lately, that I had some free time and thought I'd stop by." He and Dad enjoyed each other's company. They were good for each other. And the Holy Spirit was calling Ed to Heidi's bedside often. Heidi has a special bonding with both Dad and Ed to this day.

It was 3:30 in the afternoon—time for shift change. As Ed and Dad gave us an update on Heidi's day, Dad motioned for me to sit down on one of the sofas in the waiting room.

He gingerly began, "Vic, the doctors have talked to us quite a bit today about Heidi's condition. It's not good. Not good at all. And getting worse daily. We all know how we want this to turn out. We've all done our part. We have prayed and fasted. But we don't *demand* of God. The final answer is in His hands. And we're all concerned about what's going to happen to you if it doesn't turn out the way we want. You've got to release her. You've got to prepare yourself for the possibility that she might not make it. We're afraid you're going to crash otherwise."

I felt his tender concern. I knew he was spending hours in prayer for her each day. Throughout my childhood, I had seen him on his knees in the family room praying every morning. It had been a silent witness which spoke volumes to me.

Heidi had wrapped her tiny fingers around his heart as he sat with her each day. He held her hand for hours. He loved her dearly. But he was also trying to help his daughter, as well as his grandchild. He and Ed had just been through eight and one-half hours of seeing Heidi and hearing the medical community's report. And it looked overwhelmingly bad!

"Dad, I do recognize how sick she is. I really do. But I also know what God has told me about her. You are asking me to prepare myself for her death. And I will not. As long as there is breath within her, I will never give up hope. It may sound like demanding to you. But within me, it's standing. I *know* what God has told me about her. And I will not give up on that. *If* I'm wrong—if I've missed hearing Him somewhere on this—and I don't believe I have—but *if* I'm wrong, then God will carry me through the time when Heidi goes to be with Him, whether it's at nineteen days, nineteen years, or ninety years. But I will *not* prepare myself for her to die."

There was that word "release" again. Dad had just used it. I had been grappling with it for over a week now. Burtis and Winifred had used it recently. Their first child had died at eleven months old. We had listened quietly in our living room one evening as they encouraged us to release Heidi to Jesus.

I didn't like that word. It made me think of giving up. And I wasn't willing to do that. I felt as if I was now getting the Christian community's version of the Reality Campaign. Release, release, release. *God, are you trying to say something to me through these people?*

In my praying, I had also been grappling with how and when the change would take place in Heidi's condition. Why was it taking so long? I felt like God's answer was: "You have believed Me, that I'm going to heal her. Now that you believe Me, sit down and wait. I will do it *when* I do it and *how* I choose to do it. It won't be late. But it will be *My Way*. So stop trying to figure Me out, like guessing when and how I'm going to do it. I know you believe Me for what, but you must also believe Me for when and how." How did the word "release" figure into all of this?

Dr. Smith's notes that day reflected what he had told Dad earlier:

> Prognosis remains very poor, and chances for survival are decreasing, as time goes on. No good surgical option. Parents desire to maintain medically for thirty days and then decide with regards to surgery. Cardiology desires to try [to take] off prostaglandin tomorrow.

Around ten o'clock that night as Heidi slept in my arms, a lady dressed in a casual pants outfit approached Chuck and me. "I'm Nancy

Dambro. I'm a pulmonologist—a lung specialist. Dr. Smith and Dr. Lai have asked me to take a look at Heidi. They wanted my input on what might be causing her lungs to collapse. I know they're also concerned about how we can get her off the respirator."

"I'm Chuck, and this is my wife Vickie. It will take us a few minutes to transfer Heidi and the tubes back to her bed so you can examine her," he explained.

"Oh, no. She's sleeping so well in your arms. Don't move. I don't want to disturb her. I'm a mother as well. You never wake a sleeping baby unless absolutely necessary. I'll listen to as much of her airway sounds as possible with her in your arms, and then do a complete check-up tomorrow."

With those words, Dr. Dambro won my heart. She was a commanding presence and a respected expert in her field of medicine. Combined with that was a mother's heart. What an unbeatable combination! Her deep voice spoke with authority on medical issues. And yet, the next minute, we were comparing stories about Sterling and her twenty-one-month-old Mary.

When she left half an hour later, Chuck glanced over at me, still holding a sleeping Heidi. "I like Dr. Dambro. I'm glad she's a part of our team of doctors. God has been placing each doctor on Heidi's team. He has a purpose for each one—in Heidi's life and in that doctor's life as well. It's going to be interesting to see what He does with all of this."

When Chuck and I arrived home late that night, I tiptoed upstairs to Sterling's crib for a midnight kiss. In the dim light, he looked like an angel with his tousled blond hair and blue footie pajamas. I missed reading to him and putting him to bed each night, even though I knew he was loving the special times with his grandparents. How many more nights would I be torn between a child at the hospital and a child at home?

As I turned to leave his room, I glanced at the picture above his crib.

"The Good Shepherd." It's a beautiful, pastoral scene. Jesus is walking through a grassy meadow surrounded by sheep. In the background, the mountains slope downward to a cool stream of water. In his right hand, Jesus carries a shepherd's staff. Cradled in His left arm is a tiny lamb looking at Him with eyes of complete trust. The look of compassion in His eyes and His protective hold on the lamb speak volumes. My thoughts returned to the "release" conversations. Could that tiny lamb be Heidi? Could I place her in Jesus' arms for Him to care for her? Yes. Release her? No, I still didn't like that word. Place her in His arms? Yes, that I could do. This was the picture I needed. Heidi was His lamb, protected in His arms. Her song, "Masterpiece," had even referred to her as a "little lamb of God."

Wednesday, December 11 — The next morning I told Adrienne about the lamb picture in our phone conversation. She had seen the same picture in a local Christian bookstore recently and offered to get one to hang at Heidi's bedside. Several hours later, when she stopped by the house she was beaming.

"I got the largest one they had. We want to make a statement of Who is in control at her bedside," she said as she held up the 16 x 20 inch framed print. "And look at this picture, Vickie. Notice the sheep around Jesus. Tell me which one is you."

I hadn't noticed the other sheep the night before. But with one glance I knew. "Why I'm the one closest to Jesus, looking up at Him and the baby lamb. Chuck is the strong one out in front with the horns, protectively looking around. I love it!"

Yes, I could place her in Jesus' arms. But that didn't mean releasing her and walking away. I was right at their side, continually focused on Jesus and my baby lamb. Once again He had given me a visual picture of what was happening in the spiritual realm.

When we arrived at the hospital that afternoon, Chuck's boss Marge was waiting for us with a Catholic priest. Marge is an American Airlines executive originally from New York whose life had been radically changed by a trip to Medjugorje several years earlier. This small village is nestled in the mountains of the former Yugoslavia. Since 1981 the Blessed Virgin Mary, the Mother of God, has allegedly been appearing to six children.

On an earlier visit to Heidi's bedside, Marge had brought holy water from Medjugorje to anoint Heidi for healing. She and her rosary group had faithfully prayed for her daily. Her concern extended beyond that of an employer to that of a sister in the Lord. She had arranged for Father Mendoza to conduct a healing service at Heidi's bedside. This short stocky man was wearing a white robe with a colorful embroidered stole. There was a no-nonsense air about him, and his strong Filipino accent forced you to listen closely to catch each word. His gifting was in the healing ministry.

Another stretch for me in my comfort zone? Yes. But was I open? YES. I didn't care what branch or branches of the Christian body God wanted to use to heal my daughter. Just do it. When you're desperate, you become much more open!

As the four of us entered the NICU, Chuck was summoned to a telephone call with Dr. Lai. As soon as he returned to her bedside, Father Mendoza began the healing service. I had always pictured Catholic worship as high church, possibly in another language, very formal and impersonal. Here I was at my first service, one of only five people. It was impossible to fade into the background. I had been concerned about not knowing what to do or how to respond at certain points. Yet what we experienced that day was an intimate sharing with another branch of the Body of Christ as we interceded for our daughter's life. We felt the sweet presence of the Holy Spirit during that prayer time. Many of the Scriptures he read were ones we were already claiming. But there were several new ones, especially Ezekiel 36:26 which promises, "Moreover, I will give you a new heart and put a new spirit within you." (NASB) Father Mendoza anointed Heidi with holy water brought from Medjugorje.

There was a special circle of Catholic believers who faithfully stood with us throughout the battle in prayer—Joe and Marge, Father Mendoza, Wade and Kae, Adrian and Mary, our neighbors Charlie and Laurie, and the rosary group. As Father Mendoza and Marge left Heidi's bedside they left behind two things: a sweet presence of the Holy Spirit and instructions to anoint Heidi daily with the bottle of Medjugorje holy water. They also left behind a stretched, more open believer—me.

"Why, I understood everything he was doing and saying," I explained to Chuck. "Didn't you? Except for when he talked really fast with his accent. That was a powerful time of prayer!"

Several minutes later, I remembered the earlier phone call from Dr. Lai. "How was your talk with Dr. Lai?" I asked, not really wanting to shift back into the medical side yet.

"I don't think you want to know," he replied.

"You know what? I *don't* want to know!" It was the first time I had responded in that way. But it was the truth. I didn't want to hear any more medical reports right then. I had had enough. Later.

For the next two hours we watched Heidi cry and struggle. Pastor Jim stopped by to pray and visit. When Chuck walked him back to the waiting room, my tears joined with Heidi's. She was fighting the tubes, fighting to breathe with partially collapsed lungs, fighting large amounts of mucous in her airways—**fighting!**

God, I cried, *I don't doubt at all that you're healing her. But how much more does she have to go through? She is suffering!*

The song He ministered to me at that moment was "For Those Tears

I Died"—"*I felt every tear drop when in darkness you cried, and I strove to remind you that for those tears I died.*"[5]

That night God sent another branch of the Body—Steve and Diane Solomon. Steve has a strong ministry of intercession through his nightly radio program "Praise in the Night." Pastor Jim had mentioned the program, but my initial thoughts had been similar to those regarding Gloria's video. *Not now. We're in survival mode. Not interested in a radio program. Especially one from eleven p.m. to six a.m.!*

Steve is an outgoing guy—a mover and a shaker—bold in the things of the Lord. The word "shy" isn't in his vocabulary! God's cast of characters is such a diverse group! He and Diane weren't intimidated at all by the medical reports. Healing was nothing new to them—just another of the wonderful things they had seen God do many times. Nightly they received reports of healings during Steve's seven hours of praise and intercession on the radio. And yet our conversation was tempered with compassion as they shared the story of a daughter who lived for six painful months before her death due to a rare chromosomal disorder. Their ministry to us was precious because they had been where we were.

As we drove through the darkened streets of downtown Fort Worth around midnight, we turned on "Praise in the Night." The first thing we heard was a song which we knew was for us:

> *He is able, more than able*
> *To accomplish what concerns me today.*
> *He is able, more than able*
> *To handle anything that comes my way.*
> *He is able, more than able*
> *To do much more than I could ever dream.*
> *He is able, more than able*
> *To make me what He wants me to be.*[6]

We then heard Steve's familiar voice telling Heidi's story and asking for prayer. It was the first of many nights of nationwide intercession on her behalf via the radio. Soon Steve even referred to her as "Heidi Praise-in-the-Night Watson."

"She's part ours, you know. We prayed for her for so long," he later teased.

It was 1:00 a.m. when we wearily climbed into bed. Just before turning off the nightstand lamp, I looked into Chuck's eyes and said, "It's okay. You can tell me what Dr. Lai said now. I'm ready."

"Are you sure?" he wondered. "It's not good."

"Yes. I'm ready."

"They are doing a bronchoscopy on Heidi tomorrow morning. They will take a scope down her respirator tube and look at her lungs. It should be fairly simple since there is a tube already in place for them to use," he explained.

"That doesn't sound too bad," I interjected.

"But the reason they're doing the test is that they think her heart may have been enlarged throughout the entire pregnancy. The breathing system may have never developed. So even if her heart were fixed, she may not have a breathing system. And there's nothing that could be done about that. We've all been concerned about the heart, but if her breathing apparatus never developed, then it doesn't even matter whether her heart is okay. None of this would ever work," he quietly concluded.

"That's a lie!" I exclaimed sitting up in bed. "Heidi *does* have a breathing system!"

"I'm just telling you what they said, honey." He sounded so tired.

"I'm not angry at you. And I'm sorry that you had to carry this news alone for nine hours. But that is a lie from the pit of hell! I'm angry at Satan. That's a last ditch flare from him! And I don't believe it!" I responded, giving my pillow a hard punch before laying my head down for the night.

Thursday, December 12 — Dr. Dambro gave us the report from the bronchoscopy at eleven o'clock that morning. Heidi's breathing system was completely normal! The breathing problems were being caused by her enlarged heart pressing on her lungs. If the heart would stop pressing on the lungs, and if she could come off the respirator, she should be able to cough up the mucous.

Past another detour. Now back to the heart! At noon that day, Dr. Lai recorded the following notes:

> Results of bronchoscopy very helpful. As per Dr. Dambro, Heidi has extrinsic compression of right bronchi from large heart. No mucous plugs seen. Findings make it unlikely for Heidi to tolerate extubation [coming off the respirator]. Would suggest that Heidi's only chance for survival would be with cardiac surgery or transplantation to reduce heart size. Spoke with Dr. Ring in Dallas regarding transplant option. Feel Heidi is presently without any permanent damage to other organ systems. Will urge parents to consider transplant and to be evaluated for such now . . . Will also try discontinuing prostaglandin in morning.

That night we experienced another tough evening with Heidi. She turned blue. Her breathing was so difficult that they replaced the respirator tube in hopes it would correct the problem. It didn't. Her blood gases, which measure the carbon dioxide level in the body, soared up to 117. They should be below 45. The nurses notified the doctor on call who rushed to her bedside.

"What does this mean?" Chuck asked.

Slowly the doctor responded, "Well, we're saying that we only have hours or days left, not weeks."

Chuck headed to the waiting room to call the prayer chain. During that time, Heidi turned blue again, and they kicked me out while they frantically worked on her. When we were allowed to return several hours later, she was peaceful and not as blue. The respirator rate was at 45—the highest yet. We were grateful to have made it through another crisis, but disappointed that the turnaround had come because of increasing the respirator rate. When would the change come because of a miracle?

Friday, December 13 — Chuck and I had discussed whether to go to the hospital that morning since they would be taking her off the prostaglandin. They would not allow us in the room during the initial period, so we decided that we could pray just as well from home and the office. Dad would be at her side as much as possible. He and the doctors would keep us updated by phone.

Our wish? That the heart duct would close and the blood would start flowing forward through her heart. That would be our miracle. If the blood did not flow through her tricuspid valve, they would have to restart the medicine. How would they track the progress? If Heidi turned blue and her oxygen levels went down, it would be an indication that she could not tolerate it.

At eleven o'clock that morning Dr. Lai telephoned to let us know they were getting ready to stop the prostaglandin. I conferenced in Chuck at the office.

Dr. Lai explained what was happening. "We'll be taking off the medication in the next half hour. We don't know how long it will take for the duct to close. It could be minutes or days. What we hope for is a gradual closing over a period of days. That would give her the best chance of handling it. But we have no idea how her duct will respond. We'll keep you posted. And we'll let your Dad come back in the room as soon as we see how things are going. Do you have any questions?"

"Dr. Lai, I have one," I responded. "This is in no way life threatening, is it? I mean, if she can't handle it, we just restart the medicine. Then we'll try again later, right?"

"Mrs. Watson, I'm glad you asked that. This is *very* life threatening. If that duct closes suddenly, we don't get a chance to reopen it. If it closes gradually, and we see that she's not handling it, there may be a window of opportunity to restart the medicine. But there are no guarantees that it will work at this point. This is a very risky thing that we are doing. But she has to come off of this medicine. She has been on it for two and one-half weeks, far longer than we would choose. We are running out of options. *Yes*, this is very life threatening."

Chuck concluded the conversation, knowing that Dr. Lai's words had probably done me in. He was right. After Dr. Lai was off the phone line, Chuck and I then talked and prayed together for a few minutes.

Our mothers were both sleeping upstairs, but had asked that I let them know when the call came. At each of their bedroom doors, I briefly explained, "Dr. Lai just called and they're getting ready to stop the medicine." I didn't walk through the rest of the conversation. They already knew anyway. I was the last family member to accept how life-threatening this could be.

It was a strange day. Very little conversation around the house. Yet we all jumped each time the phone rang. Everyone froze to see if it was the hospital.

Dad called around 12:30 with a report. "It doesn't appear there's anything different since they removed the prostaglandin, so that's good news."

For once, no change in her condition was welcomed news. Chuck and I were encouraged by what we saw when we arrived at her bedside late that afternoon. Her oxygen saturation levels were stable. She seemed peaceful—no signs of frustration or pain. She had even opened her eyes and looked at Grandpa several hours earlier.

Dr. Lai's notes on the medical chart at 5:30 p.m. sounded equally encouraging:

> Child off prostaglandin, past seven hours. But PDA [duct] still open—evident by oxygen saturation levels in 90's. Will re-echo [echocardiogram] if oxygen sats drop into 70's to assess pulmonic and tricuspid valves as PDA closes. Spoke to Dr. Leonard, surgeon at Dallas Children's Hospital. Their feeling is that radical surgery to oversew tricuspid valve should not be offered there.

Chuck called Pat with an update at 8:00 that night:

Pat: "Well, you sound chipper. How's our baby?"

Chuck: "Our baby has been off the medicine now since 11:30 a.m. So far she's doing good. The doctor doesn't think the duct has closed yet. We tell him that we think it has closed, and the blood is flowing in the right direction. We think we have our miracle! He doesn't think enough hours or days have passed yet, because so far all the oxygen sats [saturation levels] have stayed up. He thinks that when the duct closes, the sats will go down . . ."

Pat: "Well, I'm with you, bud! Can they do a sonogram or something to see if the duct is open or shut?"

Chuck: "We asked them that, but the sonogram people are off for the weekend."

Pat: "UGHHHHHHH!"

Chuck: "My immediate response was the same as yours. You know, I was frustrated. Then I thought, 'Well now, God knew that. He's in control. God knew they were going to do this on a Friday and that they're off on the weekend.' But I felt like you did, you know. My human part was just frustrated."

Pat: "... Well, by Monday we'll know for sure."

Chuck: "That's right."

Pat: "They won't even need the sonogram."

Chuck: "My concern was if something else were to go wrong with Heidi. I don't want them to put her back on the medicine thinking that's the problem, when that's not the problem at all. You know what I'm saying?"

Pat: "Yes. Exactly."

Chuck: "But God is all-knowing, and He's in control. So I've got to trust Him with that too."

Pat: "That's right. I really feel like if something were going to happen, it would have happened shortly after they took her off that medicine. God is in complete control of this, and His timing is perfect. When she was ready to come off of all that, He told them to take her off. He knows what's going on ... I talked to Carol, my prayer partner, this morning. By the time I finally got hold of her, it was about 11:20 to 11:45 and I said that Heidi had already been off the medication for some time. As it turned out, our prayer was right when it was happening. In a vision, Carol saw the Lord touching Heidi's heart. Then she had another vision right after that of His hand just laying across her chest. And she saw little baby angels surrounding her bed, just kinda hovering and surrounding her, and singing praises to the Lord. And the blood was flowing freely through her heart. It was wonderful."

Chuck: "Praise the Lord! Her coloring is back, so I just praise the Lord for that. If that's the sign that confirms that it has happened—I don't know. But I'm thanking God for healing!"

Pat: "Really! Absolutely! . . . As we were praying, she had a word from the Lord. *She will not turn blue. Her blood is flowing freely. Her lungs are filling with air.* And she was speaking to her lungs and saying, 'Take another breath, Heidi, of pure unadulterated air. Just breathe deeply.' She will not turn blue."

Chuck: "Did she have any Scripture?"

Pat: "Yes. Ezekiel 37 where it was talking about the dead bones: *Thus saith the Lord God unto these bones; Behold, I will cause breath to enter into you, and ye shall live: And I will lay sinews upon you, and will bring up flesh upon you, and cover you with skin, and put breath in you, and ye shall live; and ye shall know that I am the Lord. So I prophesied as I was commanded: and as I prophesied, there was a noise, and behold a shaking, and the bones came together, bone to his bone. And when I beheld, lo, the sinews and the flesh came up upon them, and the skin covered them above: but there was no breath in them. Then said he unto me, Prophesy unto the wind, prophesy, son of man, and say to the wind, Thus saith the Lord God; Come from the four winds, O breath, and breathe upon these slain, that they may live. So I prophesied as he commanded me, and the breath came into them, and they lived, and stood up upon their feet, an exceeding great army.* (Ezekiel 37:5-10, KJV) We read that together . . . and she was prophesying it over Heidi. It was awesome!"

Chuck: "Well, praise the Lord! We receive it!"

Pat: "Amen. And I transferred our prayer time onto the tapes I'm recording of our conversations. We're on the second side of tape two now."

Chuck: "It's like a book, isn't it! Vickie says the name of the book is *Miracle Heidi.*"

Pat: "It's going to be really neat to listen to the tapes from beginning to end, from day one to the day—we'll end it with her dedication ceremony on tape. That'll be wonderful."

Chuck: "A week from Sunday. It's a week from Sunday."

Pat: "I know! The last prophecy she had last week was that He was healing her in stages. This is another stage. When Dr. Dambro did the lung test, her breathing was normal. That was a stage. Now today, this is another stage . . . we just saw her whole and well in a vision . . . every ministry I've called, every prayer counselor I've called to pray, they get the same word . . . *'This baby is to live and shall not die!!!'* Every single one without fail has said the same thing. It's just like pushing play on the recorder and they all say the same thing . . . I can't wait for her to have the final victory and be TOTALLY healed. I can't wait??? What am I saying? Who am I to say that? What a testimony this baby is going to have—all over the world."

Chuck: "And I believe that other people will be brought to God because of her."

Pat: "Oh, I do too. When people have been made aware of her and then the word goes out that her miracle has come and she's totally whole—it is going to be a testimony to a lot of people. Well, you give Vickie my love . . ."

Chuck: "If we have any new developments, we'll let you know. We love you."

Pat: "Bless you. Bye."

Chapter Nine

On Stage—Heidi

Saturday, December 14 — During the day Heidi's oxygen sats dropped from the 90's to the 80's, and her carbon dioxide levels were elevated slightly.

Mother's journal reflected the tone of the entire family throughout that day: "Nurse Laurie said the heart duct is closing. It's scary." We were walking on egg shells, yet hopeful.

Sunday, December 15 — Chuck stayed with Heidi that morning so Mother and Dad could attend church together and watch Jeremy and Jessica perform in the Christmas play. I went with them. It was exciting to stand and finally report good news to this congregation who had interceded so faithfully. When I announced that Heidi was off the heart medicine, they applauded.

But when I returned to the hospital that afternoon, it was obvious that things were headed downhill once again. Her carbon dioxide levels were increasing. X-rays showed more collapsed areas in her lungs. The respirator settings had been turned back up. She was back on 100% oxygen, and her oxygen sats were down into the 70's.

As I left the room in tears, one of our nurses walked over to Chuck and said, "If it means anything to you, every nurse in this place is pulling for Heidi."

It was 9:00 p.m. I called home and the prayer chain. It was difficult even repeating the nurse's words—congestive heart failure—as we sent forth yet another plea for prayer. I then fled to the prayer chapel. I felt as if I had been slapped in the face for daring to report good news that morning at church. After the flood of tears subsided, I turned to the Psalms hoping for something to soothe the weary aching of my own heart. Many times I had skimmed over the "pit Psalms"—the depressing ones written in the pits. But tonight they vividly expressed my journey. *God, I know where he was when he wrote this.*

Psalms 42 and 43 were for me:

> . . . My tears have been my food day and night, While they say to me all day long, "Where is your God?" These things I remember, and I pour out my soul within me. For I used to go along with the throng and lead them in procession to the house of God, With the voice of joy and thanksgiving, a multitude keeping festival . . . O my God, my soul is in despair within me . . . All Thy breakers and Thy waves have rolled over me . . . I will say to God my rock, "Why hast Thou forgotten me? Why do I go mourning because of the oppression of the enemy?" As a shattering of my bones, my adversaries revile me, While they say to me all day long, "Where is your God?" . . . Vindicate me, O God, and plead my case against an ungodly nation; . . . For Thou art the God of my strength; why hast Thou rejected me? Why do I go mourning because of the oppression of the enemy? O send out Thy light and Thy truth, let them lead me; Let them bring me to Thy holy hill, And to Thy dwelling places. Then I will go to the altar of God, To God my exceeding joy; And upon the lyre I shall praise Thee, O God, my God. Why are you in despair, O my soul? And why are you disturbed within me? Hope in God, for I

shall again praise Him, The help of my countenance, and my God. (NASB)

God, I do need Your Light and Your Truth, because I certainly don't understand what's going on. Nothing was fitting together. I was painfully aware that we had now entered the time frame of December 14-22. Remember the sign: "On Stage—Heidi, December 14-22." Congestive heart failure was not my idea of being on stage!

I went back to her bedside and played the tape I had made for her that first week of her life—more for my benefit than for Heidi's. It was 10:30 p.m. How I wanted to hold my baby, but I knew she wasn't doing well. There was no way they would let me hold her on a rough night like this.

As I sat down, Chuck walked over with Lisa our nurse. "Would you like to hold her?" she asked.

I couldn't believe my ears. "I would love to, but I know she is in such distress right now."

"You know, we have to move her to weigh her anyway. And we feel as if you should hold her," Lisa replied.

What a mixture of emotions! I was thrilled to hold her and yet thinking, *Lord, I'll probably just sit here and cry all over her.* The tears were right at the surface.

Her oxygen sats had been in the 70's, 60's, 50's, down to 49. Within three minutes of being placed in my arms, her sats went into the 80's and stayed between 78 and 91. I sat amazed. Such a peace came over her and then over me when they placed her in my arms. I held her for almost four hours—until 2:15 a.m.

As I shared the experience with Pat on the phone the next day, there was another interesting side to what was happening in prayer during those moments:

Pat: "Carol and I prayed for Chuck and you last night—separately . . . There was a lot of weariness in you. This was probably about the time you had left the chapel and gone in to be with her. We asked for supernatural strength to flow through you into Heidi. We asked that the nurses would let you hold her. And that your anointing (that was given you last Sunday night when we prayed for you) would be refreshed and would flow through you as healing."

Vickie: "You know, I didn't realize that was what was happening at the time until one of my friends came in late last night. Out in the waiting room, Chuck had told her what had happened and how Heidi had incredibly improved when I held her . . . and she said, 'Vickie, that's the healing power flowing through you.' It took her saying that for me to click back to that. It was a lesson for me too. Because when I went in there, I was so low. I was even concerned that Heidi would pick up on that. That's why I was reluctant to hold her even though I felt like I was supposed to. So when my friend said that, I thought, 'God, I know that was all totally You and not an ounce of me, because there wasn't any of me left in there.' I feel like He was teaching me and saying, 'When you least expect it is when I can work through you.'"

Pat: "Exactly! And that anointing is always on you. Whether you *feel* it or not. That doesn't matter. It's still there. So every time you touch her, that healing anointing flows through you . . ."

Vickie: "Last night it was incredible to watch what the nurses started doing. [They have never had a family stay at the bedside around-the-clock like this before in the NICU. And there are many restrictions concerning what can and can't be done in there.] They wouldn't let us have drinks. They're very particular about everything. Well, when Heidi got settled in my arms and her sats went back up, all the nurses kept coming over and saying, 'I've never seen her like this' . . . They said they were going to do the breathing treatments with her in my arms. 'You can do that?' I questioned. She said, 'We'll do anything we can with her in your arms right now.' They completely skipped one breathing treatment after having gone from every 15-20 minutes of doing them. She said, 'I'm going to get you some ice water and a pillow for your back and a stool for your feet . . . You tell me whatever you need. This is working. And we will do whatever works.'"

Pat: "Great! . . . Carol and I were praying for the nurses last night after you called . . . for their steps to be ordered by the Lord rather than by medical means. That they would not do what they would do normally, medically speaking, but only what the Holy Spirit told them to do . . . every hand that would touch her, that He would speak to them individually and cause them to do what God wanted done in Heidi."

Vickie: "Wow! Did He ever! . . . It was like they could not do enough for us last night. At one time, the nurse came over and said it was time for her morphine, time for her breathing treatment, time for her dressing to be changed. 'She looks real comfortable to me. What do you think?' I said, 'I think she's doing great.' She replied, 'Let's not do any of that stuff.' I'll tell you what, your *specific* prayers . . ."

Pat: "Yeah, and they were very specific . . . I'm sure other people that you had called were praying the same way. So, it's that combined prayer."

At midnight Mother joined me at Heidi's bedside while Chuck napped and visited with his mother out in the waiting room. Mother was surprised at the change in Heidi since seven-thirty p.m. when I had called the house for prayer. We enjoyed the quiet time together. Dad and she had never stayed with us for this length of time before and yet we had seen very little of each other. We had been like ships passing in the night for the three and one-half weeks since Heidi's birth, communicating more by notes and phone calls than in person although living in the same house. When she was sleeping, I was taking care of Sterling. When she was with Heidi, I was sleeping. And when she was taking care of Sterling, I was with Heidi.

Chuck and I knew we could not have maintained this level of care for both Heidi and Sterling without our parents' sacrificial help. They had put their lives on hold to help us. Although everyone was extremely weary, the plan seemed to be working. But none of us was sure how much longer we could hold up under this. Emotionally and physically, it was wearing!

Monday, December 16 — Monday morning's reports from the doctors held good news! Dr. Smith called early that morning with a report that the x-rays had showed her heart to be "less generous in size."

Dr. Lai called later that morning with the report from the sonogram. "The duct in her heart is so small that I can't really even tell if it's completely closed, or if it's just barely, barely open. But we can be cautiously optimistic," he informed us.

"Cautiously optimistic"—those were the most promising words we had heard come out of Dr. Lai's mouth!

As Chuck and I listened on telephone extensions in the kitchen and living room, we were stretching the phone cords so that we could see each other. Tears trickled down Chuck's cheek as he responded, "That's great news." I punched my fist upward into the air, mouthing a silent cheer of "*Yes!*"

Dr. Lai continued, "I'm obviously very pleased with what we've seen over the weekend and with what we're seeing now. I understand she had a tough time for a little while last night. But I'm pleased. Things are now going the way we would have wanted them to go all along."

"Well, we're pleased too, Dr. Lai," Chuck managed to say through his tears. "We've waited a long time to hear this kind of report."

"Yes. Now the three of us are going to sit down tomorrow as planned with Dr. Smith to discuss the next steps," he reminded us. When that meeting was originally set up at the end of last week, it was for them to press us to decide where to send her as a last resort—probably Dallas for a heart transplant. We had been dreading it.

Dr. Lai continued, "I would assume that probably all agree that we should follow the same course. We're getting more aggressive on bringing her off the respirator. So what we need to do is continue to—" And then he stopped.

"So, Dr. Lai," I interjected, "*we* need to continue to pray and *you* need to continue the medical care. Right?"

"Yes, that's right," he laughed. "We're doing our part, and you're doing your part."

It was a welcome change—ending a medical report on a light-hearted note.

Late that night, Dr. Dambro noted on Heidi's chart that she seemed to be doing well off the prostaglandin. Her heart size was down, and there were fewer collapsed areas in her lungs. It appeared that we had weathered the closing of the heart ductus.

Tuesday, December 17— My day started at Dr. Mann's office. This time, it was Sterling. He had a croupy night so I spent the morning in the pediatrician's office and the x-ray lab.

My emotions were near the surface by the time Sterling and I got to the x-ray stage. They were as gentle as you can be when you're trying to get a twenty-two-month-old boy to lie face down on a cold metal table without moving. Finally the technician looked at me in desperation and said, "You're just going to have to lie across his body to hold him still." I used all my strength to hold him down. He was screaming. And by this time, the tears were streaming down my face. *God, how much more for my children? How much more will they have to suffer? And how much more do I have to watch them go through?* I never dreamed that being a mother could bring such pain.

Sterling had bronchitis and an upper respiratory infection with lots of congestion. After getting his prescriptions filled, I settled him in at home with his grandmothers.

Heidi's nurse had called to remind us of our noon meeting with the doctors. She also mentioned that the IV in Heidi's arm was not working. They still had the central line which had been inserted surgically. But the prostaglandin could not be put through the central line if it should have to be restarted in an emergency. They had to have an IV line through which no other medications had passed. And finding an open vein in Heidi was a slow, tedious process. One night Chuck had tearfully watched the nurses try fifteen times before they were successful. An emergency would not allow for that kind of time. The only option left would be to put an IV in her head, which they didn't want to do. Neither did we. I had witnessed this before. It was not a pretty sight. Thus began another yo-yo day of ups and downs. Although so far there had mostly been downs.

There were five of us present for the meeting—Dr. Lai, Dr. Smith, Dad, Chuck, and me. This time we found ourselves in a different conference room in the maze of hallways near the NICU, seated around a wooden table. That was fine with me. The room where we usually met held painful memories. Maybe this was to be a new beginning. Maybe this conference would actually yield positive news!

We were a comfortable group by now—having interacted almost daily over the past twenty-seven days. They knew every member of our family well. Understood us? No, I don't think they would ever totally understand where we were coming from. But they pretty well knew what to expect from us by now. Total involvement at her bedside and in all medical decisions. And we knew what to expect from them. Excellent medical care but little encouraging news.

Chuck had summed it up well in a recent talk with Dr. Lai. "We view Heidi's care as being in the hands of a team consisting of her doctors, nurses, and family. That care involves three areas. The hospital team is responsible for the *medical* part. We her family and friends are responsible for the *spiritual and emotional* arenas. That is why we are at her side twenty-four hours a day, holding her hand, touching her, singing to her, and praying. We're also trying to make the good touching outweigh the painful touching that she receives." Dr. Lai had seemed comfortable with that division of labor.

At the beginning of the conference, Chuck mentioned our concern about Heidi being given morphine by some nurses regardless of her condition. "*If* she needs it—that is, if she appears to be in pain or distress, then we're not opposed to it. We want her to be as comfortable as possible. But there are times when she's sleeping peacefully or calmly interacting with one of us, and a nurse, especially Katie will bring morphine. We'd like her to receive it only when it's obvious that there is a need for it," explained Chuck.

"We have no problem with that," replied Dr. Smith. "We can simply make a note in her chart that it is no longer to be given on a schedule, but on an as-needed basis. I sense there may have been a problem with Katie. Do we need to do something there?"

"Well, she frequently asks us not to touch Heidi. I think all of the staff here know us well enough by now to know that we're not going to do anything that is detrimental to Heidi. We're here with her twenty-four hours a day, and we are very aware of what helps her and what doesn't. We read her signals clearly. You know that we're not going to be touching her unless it's helping her," said Chuck.

"Oh, your family's touching and holding of Heidi have been extremely beneficial. Over and over, we've watched her heart rate and breathing improve when you're holding her. There's no question about that," replied Dr. Smith. "Well, are you asking me to pull Katie off the case? I will do it. She is a good nurse. But you need to feel comfortable with whoever is caring for your daughter."

"Technically we have no questions about her ability. We feel that Heidi has received excellent care from every doctor and nurse here. We're grateful for everything that has been done for her. She has received the best care available. We're just trying to work through this Katie issue," responded Chuck.

"Well, if you're asking me to pull her off, I will," offered Dr. Smith.

"My first thought is that it would be easier," said Chuck glancing my way. He knew how difficult this one had been for me on top of everything else.

There was a struggle going on within me at that moment. Katie was a tough one for me to handle emotionally. She had brought me to tears with our "how do you think your daughter is doing" conversation and the "how is your marriage" check-up. I was uneasy around her and knew there was a war going on within her. She had a close friend fighting a terminal illness. And here we were daring to believe for our daughter who seemed certain to be terminal. It was an uncomfortable mix between Katie and me.

But this was my daughter I was watching out for. Wasn't I supposed to do that? Couldn't we use one less hassle in our lives right now? Yet I really did believe God had placed every single doctor and nurse on Heidi's case for a purpose. We were already seeing the impact on some lives. Nurse Sarah was a favorite to every member of our family. Her boys had recently named their new dog "Heidi." When Sarah had left our Heidi's bedside on the previous Friday, she had remarked to one of the Christian nurses, "You know, I'm starting to believe that maybe there's something to all of this."

Yes, these were divine appointments for each doctor and nurse. A way for God to speak to them of His power. So who was I to rearrange His roster for my ease?

Chuck continued, "But no, I feel like we're not to pull her off the case at this point." I relaxed, knowing that this tough yet tender man was receiving his orders from God. That he was operating out of God's wisdom.

Dad breathed an audible sigh of relief. "That's wonderful. She's a good nurse," he said. Dad and Katie had spent many hours together on the day shift. I realized then that God was probably using Dad and Chuck to speak to her.

Next we focused on Heidi's condition. Our elation at her having come off prostaglandin was evident. Finally we had something to celebrate!

But that elation was short-lived. Dr. Lai's next words quickly squelched the joyous mood. "We understand your excitement at Heidi being off the heart medicine. We're all very pleased. But you need to realize that you have a daughter who is ventilator-dependent. *If* she should surprise us and make it, there is no indication that she will ever come off the respirator. That brings up the question of quality of life. Have you thought about what kind of life that would be for her? Is that fair to her? What about the impact on your family? These are serious issues you're going to be forced to deal with if she does live."

I felt as if I had just aced a test and then been told that the score did not count toward the final grade. This was our first big step in the right direction. We had waited twenty-seven days to see this! And now you're telling me that even if she should surprise you and live, she'll be hooked to this respirator for the rest of her life? That I'll forever hear this whooshing mechanical pumping when I'm with her? That I'll never hear my child laugh? That she will never run through the kitchen and leap into Chuck's arms when he arrives home from work?

But the Holy Spirit gently brought my mind back to Him. "Vickie, they are focusing on *facts*. You are to focus on *truth*—what God told you about Heidi in the months before her birth."

Quin Sherrer and Ruthanne Garlock give a clear picture of the difference between facts and truth in their book *A Woman's Guide to Spiritual Warfare*. They refer to the Bible story of Deborah in Judges chapters four and five. God used her to lead the people of Israel out of twenty long years of oppression under Jabin. "Facts and truth are not always the same! The truth was that God had promised victory in spite of the odds, if Israel would obey him. Deborah—who was called 'a mother in Israel' (Judges 5:7)—was willing to stake the nation's future on that promise . . . But she acted on God's truth, not on circumstantial facts . . . Deborah and Barak were assured of victory because they battled according to God's instructions. God would not do it for them without their effort, nor did he reveal the entire strategy in advance. They had to obey God without knowing all the reasons why."[7]

So we were to focus on the direction God was leading us. Regardless of what we heard from the medical community. And regardless of what we saw in the physical realm. And we certainly didn't understand the "why" behind our obedience to God.

Dr. Lai continued, "We are still trying to get her off the respirator as aggressively as possible. But the only option left for her survival is a heart transplant. She needs to be evaluated by the team in Dallas to see if she is even a potential candidate. And that needs to happen right away. You seem to be waiting for some miraculous change that obviously has not happened."

"I want thirty days for her here, which would be Saturday. Just give us thirty days to wait here and maintain," I pleaded.

It was what we had dreaded. Being forced into the transplant route when what we both felt was that we were to wait—at least thirty days. Surgery just did not seem to be the route God would use this time. How do you convey that to a skilled team of doctors? How do you explain why you're not jumping at the only apparent option left for your child's life?

"Then our suggestion would be to send her to Dallas next Monday the twenty-third to be evaluated for a transplant," proposed Dr. Lai.

"I talked with Dr. Ring by phone earlier this week as you had requested," said Chuck. "He leaves Monday for ten days over the Christmas holidays."

"Then there's no need to send her over there to wait. We're in a better position to gage her condition right now. We know her history. But you need to understand that she heads to Dallas January first when the team returns. That's her only hope now—a heart transplant," Dr. Lai concluded. "Any questions?"

"Yesterday you both mentioned that Heidi's heart was smaller in size," I commented. "How much smaller?"

"Well, Mrs. Watson, you need to remember that she was born with her heart as enlarged as it could possibly be. It filled the entire chest cavity and pressed against the lungs. That's what caused the persistent problem with portions of her lungs collapsing. The oxygen cannot get into the lungs because the heart is pressing against them. So we're talking about a small decrease in size. But nothing even close to normal," explained Dr. Lai.

"How much smaller?" I persisted. "Give me a number. I want to know where we are as opposed to where we need to be. If her heart needs to reduce in size by one hundred percent, where are we now?"

Hesitantly, he responded, "I would cautiously say twenty percent. I don't like to put numbers on these things. It's not that easy to be accurate. I think we could safely say that her heart size has reduced by one-fifth. But don't forget, even if it should reduce to a normal size—which will not happen—you still have a defective heart valve. The heart shrinking would help the lungs. That would be her only chance to come off the respirator. But you would still have a major valve problem. Do you have any other questions?"

"No questions. Just an invitation," said Chuck. "We'd like to invite you both to Heidi's christening at our church when she comes home."

I loved this man. He continually amazed me with these bold statements of faith, usually following strong statements of facts. Both doctors stumbled around on that one, uncomfortably mumbling yes, and quickly ending the conference.

Dr. Lai's notes outlined the plan:

> Conference held earlier with parents, grandfather, Dr. Smith, and myself attending. Child has improved in some respects since prostaglandins discontinued. Pulmonary blood flow less and heart smaller. But still with segmental lung atelectasis [collapsed areas] off and on . . . However, despite improvement thus far, more improvement necessary before child can be extubated [brought off respirator]. Parents appear to understand situation at this point. They agree to having child evaluated by Dr. Steve Ring for transplantation when Dr. Ring is available. Parents understand if Heidi becomes worse in interim, nothing else can be done.

We breathed a sigh of relief as we left the conference. A twenty percent reduction in heart size? We were thrilled! And we had bought some time. We had until January 1 before we would be pushed on the transplant issue again. Of course, it would be a mute point by then. This was the week of December 14-22. Heidi was "on stage." She was to be dedicated this Sunday morning. The doctors would have really been blown away if Chuck had mentioned that we planned to have her dedicated in five days!

That night, Chuck and I spread out our dinner on the coffee table in the waiting room. We ate at six-thirty each evening during the hour-long nurses' shift change. Every morning and evening all visitors had to leave the NICU during that one hour.

Our neighbors and Chuck's co-workers provided sack lunches which we brought to the hospital each evening. They were delicious. Submarine sandwiches . . . fresh fruit with scrumptious dip . . . marinated baked chicken. We were the blessed recipients of their creativity. Our church brought a hot meal to our home every night for the grandparents and Sterling. And we finished it off around midnight or one o'clock a.m. when we arrived home.

The waiting room had become our nightly living room. The room was empty except for us. We sat on the floor and spread our food on the circular coffee table. But that night, not even the gourmet meal lifted my spirits.

After we blessed our food, I told Chuck about Sterling's x-ray ordeal that morning. "Life is not fair, Chuck. It's just not fair," I complained.

"Vickie, we already knew that," he responded tenderly. He was good at allowing me to express my frustration without giving me a sermon, although I usually had one ready for his difficult moments!

No sooner were the words out of his mouth than the Christmas carolers came singing their way through the waiting room. I wanted to scream at them.

"Chuck, everyone is having Christmas," I accused. "I'm angry at them. How could they? How could life go on for the rest of the world while we're stuck here in this hospital? How could they possibly celebrate Christmas? How dare they!"

We ate most of our meal in silence. Chuck probably felt as if he was having dinner with Scrooge, although he certainly understood. And it was difficult to ignore the strains of music drifting our way as the carolers wandered through the halls of the hospital.

As we stuffed our trash back into the paper bag, I leaned my head over on Chuck's shoulder. "Well, honey, shall we end this pity party I started?"

"Yeah, let's end it and go in and love on Heidi!" he replied pulling me up from the floor and hugging me. What would we do without each other? God seemed to keep one of us able to encourage the other at all times. We had not hit bottom at the same time. That was something to be grateful for!

Wednesday, December 18 — Heidi had a very good day. They were able to wean the respirator rate lower and lower. By that night the doctors discussed the possibility of trying her off the respirator the next morning. If they could get the rate as low as five by morning, they would try it.

Meanwhile, at home, Sterling was very sick and not sleeping well at all. Between our parents and us, we were changing shifts from one sick child to another.

Thursday, December 19 — At seven-thirty that morning, they took Heidi off the respirator. Chuck and I arrived a few minutes later and were greeted by Sarah our nurse hugging us and saying, "It's off. We're going for it!" There was an air of expectancy all around as we raced to her bedside after a hurried less-than-thorough scrubbing in and gowning. The entire unit was aware of what was going on. They were all rooting for us.

But within minutes Heidi's distress was obvious. Sarah, who had taken care of her many times and become very close to our family, suggested that I hold her. It was day twenty-nine of her life and my first time to hear her cry since those futile attempts in the delivery room. She struggled. She looked frightened. Her coloring was dark. I felt helpless as I tried to calm her. It was so frightening, and yet I knew I needed to stay calm for her sake. But it wasn't enough. It wasn't working. We blew oxygen in her face through a tube.

Sarah hesitantly offered, "Would you like me to try?"

"Oh, please, Sarah! Whatever you think will work!" I replied as I handed her over. It wasn't going well at all. We felt so helpless seeing the fear in Heidi's eyes as she gasped for each breath. And she couldn't stop crying, which was contributing to her difficulties.

After Sarah tried in vain to soothe her, it was obvious to the doctors that something had to be done. The portable oxygen wasn't even helping. They moved to an intermediate step, CPAP. A tube was inserted down her nose to the bottom of her throat to deliver puffs of air, forcing her to breathe deeper. This is often necessary for an infant who has not done the work of breathing on her own.

Chuck left the room long enough to call for prayer. Within an hour we all had to admit that she couldn't do it. Not yet. I didn't stick around to watch the large respirator tube go back down her throat. Chuck stayed at her side while I escaped to the chapel.

Several hours later that morning, Dr. Lai noted on her chart:

> Heidi is four weeks old with Ebstein's malformed tricuspid valve. Still dependent on intubated ventilator support with failed extubation attempt . . . But now off prostaglandins with satisfactory pulmonary flow and oxygen saturation levels. Heart less enlarged with less atelectasis. Continued moderately prominent tricuspid regurgitation and congenital heart failure. Parents aware that despite recent progress child may not tolerate being

weaned from ventilator. But efforts to wean from ventilator can be repeated perhaps with steroid therapy and at different rates.

Saturday, December 21 — Throughout Friday and Saturday, I had to face the fact that Heidi would *not* be dedicated that Sunday. That nothing miraculous was going to happen in those few remaining hours. That we would not walk into church with her on Sunday morning and line up with the other proud parents cradling newborns in their arms.

I had been wrong. I had missed it. I still wasn't sure what "On Stage—Heidi" was supposed to mean for the dates December 14-22. But it was obvious it was not to be her dedication. I was disappointed on timing. That was my battlefield throughout the weekend.

Chuck and I shared my feelings with two friends who visited with us in the waiting room that evening. The husband said, "Somebody somewhere is still doing a little bit of growing through this."

My reply. "I wish I knew who it was. I would say, 'You grow fast!!'"

We had heard of phenomenal changes in the members of our church body through the intercession for Heidi. As the days had lengthened into weeks and now into a month with no major changes, many of us had our searchlights on high beam looking inward for the reason. Why had there been no breakthrough in Heidi's healing? It certainly was not from lack of prayer. Within our spiritual community, there had been a bonding through the weeks of prayer for Heidi. Confessions were common as people searched their own hearts when coming before God and asking Him to heal Heidi.

One man had sat on the sofa in our family room on a recent afternoon and confessed to Chuck his ongoing secret involvement in prostitution for years. The brokenness in this family man was evident as he tearfully admitted, "I had to tell someone and start to get this straightened out. I don't want my sin, as a member of the body, to be a blockage to our prayers for Heidi."

Another lady in our church, whom I had not met at the time, sent us a precious note saying:

> There has been a situation in my life the past two months that hasn't been right. Satan has been ripping me up over it. It has stood in the way of my relationship with God also. This week I got total freedom. I need to ask your forgiveness because I haven't been able to pray for you and Heidi Joy as I should. And the Lord has shown me this week as I have been able to get in the Word in Isaiah 59:2 (NIV): "But your iniquities have separated you from your God; your sins have hidden his face from you, so that He will not hear." The times I did pray God didn't hear my prayer because of where I was. I'm sorry if I've been a part of keeping any miracle from happening for you. I know God will hear me now. We're still believing for a miracle.

God was certainly using the situation to turn many peoples' eyes toward Him. Was He causing it? **No!** But He was causing good things to come out of the situation. And that soul-searching had been taking place within Chuck and me as well.

But there came a point for both of us when we had to say, "God, You know our hearts. We have searched and don't know anything else to do. So if there is something within either of us that is a blockage here, we have to trust You to tell us. Because we can't go through any more of the 'what ifs' about this. It's too draining emotionally."

I was now at the end of my rope. I wasn't sure what I understood or believed about healing. I did know that I did *not* understand God's timing. I didn't want any more signs—especially if there was a time line attached to them. No, don't tell me about them. Just let me know when she is healed!

Chuck was good for me that night when we returned to Heidi's bedside after dinner and the nurses' shift change. He engulfed her dainty hand within his large masculine hands and began to pray. "Jesus, I want to thank you that the prostaglandins are off now. Thank you that her heart is smaller. Thank you that she is able to take breast milk through a stomach tube . . ." And he walked through each step that we had made. I needed to be reminded of each tiny step. Yes, there had been progress. Then he went on into thanking Him for what would be forthcoming—off the respirator, fully inflated lungs, adequate feeding by mouth, a functioning tricuspid valve. I needed to hear that too.

The doctors told us they would probably try to take the respirator off again on Sunday. Dr. Smith would be on duty all day and had wanted to be there this time to monitor her progress.

"Vickie, I think we should be here at the hospital tomorrow morning," Chuck suggested. "Especially if they're going to take off the respirator. And there is no need in putting ourselves through the baby dedication at church. We're happy for those parents and wouldn't want any of them to have to go through what we're experiencing. But emotionally, it's just too much. I don't think either of us could handle it at this point." He was painfully aware that I had been crying off and on for the past twenty-four hours. My disappointment at her healing not being completed by the twenty-second was acute.

"There is one thing the pastor offered that I feel I should at least tell you about, Vickie. Pastor Jim is willing to set up closed-circuit television and dedicate her from her bedside tomorrow with the church watching on a large screen. He's aware that this has been a tough one for you."

"No," came my immediate emphatic response. "I was wrong about December 22 being her dedication day. **I was wrong.** And I have to handle that. But doing it from her bedside would be manipulating the circumstances to *make* it happen. And that's not right. When God sends a word, then He also makes it happen. I missed it on this one. And that's my problem. No, when Heidi is dedicated, it will be in person before our church body and friends. Right now I don't want to even think about when that might be."

"I thought that was what you would think," he said. "I guess we have each other figured out pretty well after seven years of marriage. And that's fine to wait. I agree with you. But I just wanted to be sure you knew about that option."

"Chuck, we haven't dared to ask what's ahead. We've just keyed in on getting her off the respirator. I know that once it's off, we're still not there. We've got to see her heart miraculously healed. I'm afraid to even ask the doctor what that means. I just keep reminding God that He said *complete healing.*"

My faith tank was nearing the empty mark. I was in the red zone where the light flashes warning you it's time to fill the tank. I had been wrong about the "On Stage—Heidi" sign. What if I was also wrong about the song and the scripture I felt He had given me during pregnancy?

As Chuck steered the van to the right, entering our subdivision at one-thirty that morning, I welcomed the soft strains of guitar music as we listened to Praise in the Night on the radio. Steve Green began to gently sing:

> *He who began a good work in you*
> *He who began a good work in you*
> *Will be faithful to complete it*
> *He'll be faithful to complete it*

He who started the work
Will be faithful to complete it in you.

As we pulled into the garage, Chuck turned off the motor but left the ignition partially on so we could hear the rest of the song:

If the struggle you're facing
Is slowly replacing your hope with despair
Or the process is long
and you're losing your song in the night
You can be sure that the Lord has His hand on you
Safe and secure, He will never abandon you
You are His treasure and He finds His pleasure in you.

He who began a good work in you
He who began a good work in you
Will be faithful to complete it
He'll be faithful to complete it
He who started the work
Will be faithful to complete it in you. [8]

Yes, the process did seem very long. And yes, I had lost my song during the last twenty-four hours of darkness. But He had just renewed it. As we sat in the darkened garage in the wee hours of that morning holding hands with tears flowing, I knew there were three of us present. My disappointment and questioning had not chased God away. Neither had my mistake about what He was saying to me. He would be faithful to complete what He had promised.

How? When? I had no idea. But for now I was to concentrate on His faithfulness.

Sunday, December 22 — Chuck and I arrived at the hospital at 7:30 that morning ready for another try at bringing her off the respirator. We had alerted the prayer chain that it would be a crucial day. Many churches would be praying that morning.

Heidi's heart rate had fluctuated throughout the night, she had some hard breathing, and her blood pressure was up. So they delayed it until 1:00 p.m. The morning was difficult, with more of what the previous night had held. She was agitated and obviously uncomfortable. Although we knew many people were praying, Chuck and I both felt an aloneness. There was a stark painful contrast between what we thought this morning was going to hold—dedication—and what we were watching Heidi experience. *God, please, at least let her come off the respirator today! Just give us this one thing!*

At 1:00 her blood pressure was too high. We would have to wait longer. At 3:30 they decided to give it a try. Dr. Smith and Dr. Dambro were both present. One of our favorite nurses Karen was Heidi's nurse for the day. Chuck and I stood at the window, a few feet away, praying fervently. We had learned to be as inconspicuous as possible at these moments. That seemed to improve our chances of staying in the room.

Even as they were getting ready to pull out the tube, Dr. Dambro repeated once again, "I don't think this is going to work. We should be bringing the respirator rate down much more slowly. We can try it, but you need to know that it's probably not going to work."

In my spirit I was saying to Heidi, *Don't believe it. Don't receive those words. You can do it, Heidi.* I couldn't wait to hold her so that I could verbalize my thoughts.

As soon as the tube was out, I picked her up and settled into the wooden rocking chair near her bed. Chuck was kneeling on the floor at my elbow. Her heart rate zoomed up to 200. She struggled and cried hard. Her coloring was bluer. It felt like an instant replay of the first attempt off the respirator. We quietly prayed over her, gently encouraged her, and sang "Jesus Loves Me" softly. Outwardly we may have appeared calm, but inwardly we were both struggling and pleading for God's mercy.

After awhile, Chuck and then Karen tried holding and calming her. When neither worked, she placed Heidi back on her bed, still struggling. I knew what the next step was, and I couldn't bear to hear it. I left her bedside in tears. Chuck remained at her side, holding her hand and praying.

Once again the chapel was my escape. I laid my head on the wooden altar across the front and sobbed. No prayers. No questions. Just painful, gut-wrenching sobs from a mother's raw heart. I didn't think I could hurt any more. And the sobs just kept coming from deep within. How long was I there? I have no idea. You become oblivious to the passing of time at those moments. But when my sobs finally began to subside, I sensed the Holy Spirit's sweet soothing presence. Nothing overwhelming. No answers. Nothing had changed. But I knew that I was not alone. That He was there with me.

I sat down on the kneeling pad of the altar, wiping away the last traces of tears and make-up. There was a pile of used tissues on the floor at my side bearing testimony to the intensity of the storm. Prayer? No, I still couldn't pray. I was too weary. And I didn't even know what I would pray at that point. Hadn't I said it all over the last month? I had no praying left within me.

It reminded me of the Bible story when Amalek fought against Israel.

> So Moses said to Joshua, "Choose men for us, and go out, fight against Amalek. Tomorrow I will station myself on the top of the hill with the staff of God in my hand." And Joshua did as Moses told him, and fought against Amalek; and Moses, Aaron, and Hur went up to

the top of the hill. So it came about when Moses held his hand up, that Israel prevailed, and when he let his hand down, Amalek prevailed. But *Moses' hands were heavy*. Then they took a stone and put it under him, and he sat on it; and Aaron and Hur supported his hands, one on one side and one on the other. Thus his hands were steady until the sun set. So Joshua overwhelmed Amalek . . . (Exodus 17:9-13, NASB)

I now understood the weariness, and yet the sense of responsibility, that Moses must have felt. There came a point when he could no longer physically hold up the staff of God in his hands. He was too weary, regardless of the consequences. I had now reached that point in my intercession for Heidi. My only hope for victory was to trust God to send people like Aaron and Hur to support my hands, to continue to pray. Because I no longer could do it.

For the first time since I had left Heidi's side, I felt an urgency to get back to her. Even as I started out of the chapel, I began to prepare myself to once again see that big blue respirator tube down her throat. How I dreaded it! She must be so weary now from the ordeal. Having to fight for each breath and not understanding why. The sound of her own cry must even be frightening after not being able to make a sound.

As I walked the now familiar long hallway back to the NICU and her bedside, the Holy Spirit gave me two words—"encourage her." By the time I reached her side, fully expecting to hear again the whooshing of the respirator, I was surprised. Holding her hand, Chuck wordlessly pointed to her mouth. Only the stomach tube for feeding remained. No respirator tube. No whooshing sound. While I was gone they had put her on CPAP, the nasal tube which delivers puffs of oxygen at the back of her throat to encourage her to breathe deeply. They were trying this as an interim step before giving up. They had also just given her valium to calm her.

Chuck took one look at my swollen red eyes and knew where I had been. He slid to the right beside Heidi's feet so that I could hold her hand. My next step was not what I would have normally done. Here was my baby exhausted and frightened. Her big eyes were pleading for help. And she continued to struggle for every breath.

I laid my head on her bed so that our eyes were only inches apart, as close as the tubes would allow. And we had a mother-daughter talk. "Heidi, we're going to do this. God has placed within you the knowledge of how to breathe. When He created you, He put that knowledge there. So you don't have to fight this. Just relax and do what Jesus is telling you to do. You *do* know how to breathe. You *can* do this. Don't give up, but relax and do what He's telling you to do. Daddy and I are here, and we will be with you all the way. It *is* going to be okay. And there will be a day when you won't have to fight to breathe. It won't always be this hard. But don't give up! Listen to Jesus. You know His voice. He's been here with you the whole time. Just do what He's telling you to do. You're going to make it!"

The rest of the day? It was long. It was a battle! But she remained off the respirator!

Pat and her husband Mike came by late in the day. It was Pat's forty-fifth birthday. She recorded her thoughts:

Mike and I went to the hospital today because I wanted to be with Heidi on my birthday! . . . I have come to love Heidi sooo much! Sometimes I feel like an intruder since I'm not family. But I feel so "bonded" to her. She is a very big and important part of my life right now . . .

I felt *so* sorry for Chuck and Vickie tonight. They are

both hurting so very much. If only there were something I could do to relieve some of *their* pain. I guess there really isn't. Vickie disappeared on us for awhile. She started to cry and got up and left . . . I looked everywhere for her and had Mike looking for her too. We thought she was going to the bathroom to "recoup" a little. But she was hurting and went outside and walked and cried out to God. Chuck was doing the same thing in the room. Inwardly he was suffering greatly as well.

The spiritual battle during this time was extremely intense!!! I could feel the intensity at times. If I had spiritually open eyes, I'm sure I would have seen quite a battle going on—literally!!

7:15 p.m. Dr. Smith's notes: "Extubated this pm and so far relatively stable on CPAP although requiring valium sedation. Will follow closely."

11:05 p.m. Dr. Smith's notes: "Stable so far on CPAP . . . Will continue on CPAP for now."

At 12:30 we finally said good night to Heidi. Our mothers had been in the waiting room for an hour, but we just couldn't bring ourselves to leave until she was sleeping.

As we climbed into the van in the parking garage, the weariness was overwhelming. So this was battle fatigue! It had been a seventeen-hour day at the hospital. And every minute of it had been war! I leaned back against the head rest and closed my eyes as we drove through the deserted streets of Fort Worth. I didn't know how Chuck could keep his eyes open to drive home. He reached over and took my hand gently.

"I don't know when we've ever been so tired, Vickie. It's been a horrendous day of battle for all of us. Harder than we would have ever dreamed. I feel like we're crawling off the battlefield. But it's from exhaustion, not defeat. And we can't lose sight of that. We won today! She has been off the respirator for nine hours now! We can't let the intensity of today, or the weariness we feel, rob us of the victory."

He was right. **We had won today!** Regardless of the fierceness of the battle, we had won this round.

And the Holy Spirit quietly placed the missing pieces in the "On Stage—Heidi, December 14-22" puzzle. What had happened during that week? Her heart ductus had closed, and she had remained off of the prostaglandins. The grand finale was her coming off the respirator on the twenty-second.

Where had the idea come from about her dedication on the twenty-second? That had come from Vickie. Yes, God had meant that sign at Bedford Boys' Ranch to be for us. But I had then placed *my* interpretation on *His* sign. When He sends His word, we are to act on it, but not to interpret it. *He* is the one who will show us what it means and how it will come to pass. It had been a painfully hard lesson for me. I had paid a dear price emotionally for interpreting His message. But He had faithfully continued to bring that which He had promised.

"On Stage—Heidi, December 14-22." Yes, indeed she was!

Photo Album

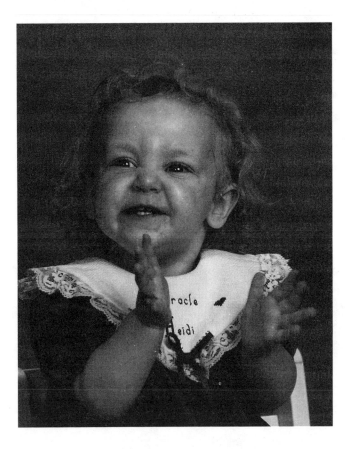

The birthday girl: "I'm one!"

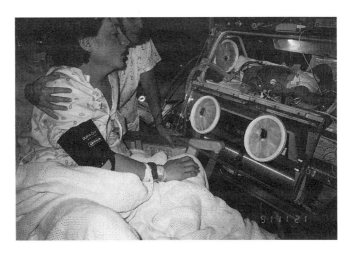

Day 1: "Take the baby to Vickie. It may be her only chance to see her alive," said the doctor.

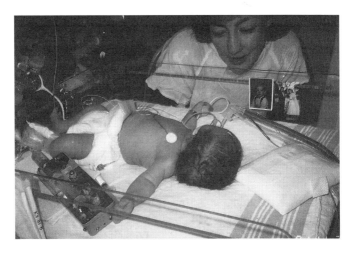

Day 4: "Heidi Joy, God says that you are a masterpiece."

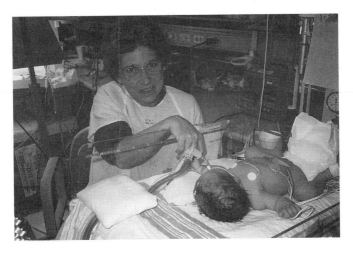

Day 5: Grandma Watson and Heidi.

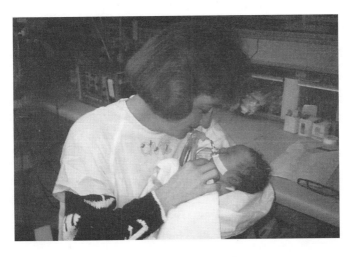

Day 10: First time in Mommy's arms.

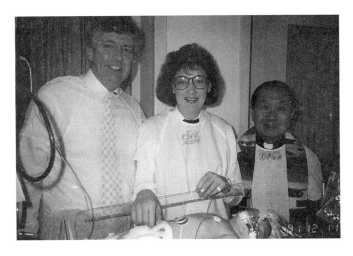

Day 21: Father Mendoza prayed at Heidi's bedside.

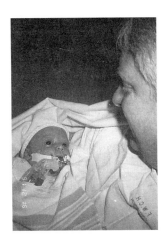

Day 26: Snuggled in Daddy's arms.

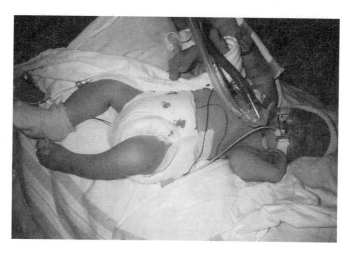

Day 26: Eleven tubes and wires connected Heidi to life support and monitors.

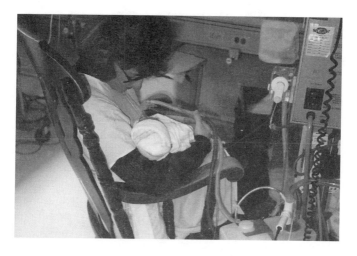

Day 30: Rocking always improved Heidi's vital signs.

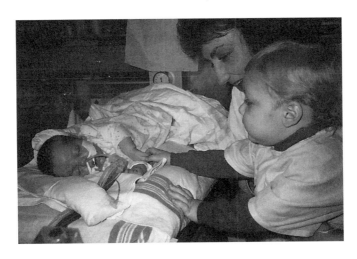

Day 34: Sterling gets acquainted with his sister on Christmas Eve. (Note Heidi's coloring—purple—from lack of oxygen.)

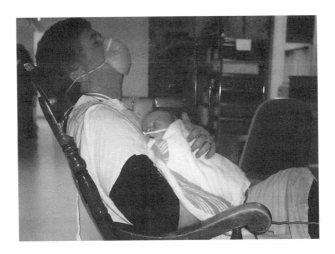

Day 41: New Year's Eve — a battle-weary father and daughter rock in the new year.

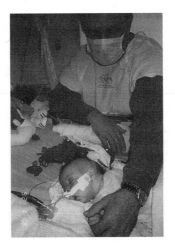

Day 54: "Grandpa" Ed and Heidi.

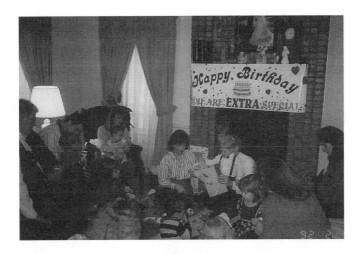

Day 74: Life goes on. Sterling's second birthday celebration.

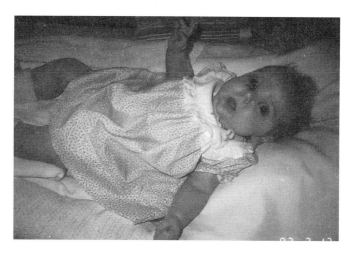

Day 84: "I'm heading out of here tomorrow!"

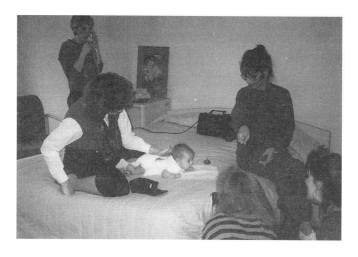

Day 85: Respiratory therapists visited us in "rooming in" to take photos and say good-bye. Intercessor Pat directs the photo session!

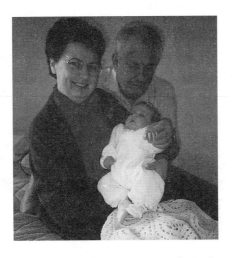

Grandma and Grandpa Boone with Heidi —
ready to go home.

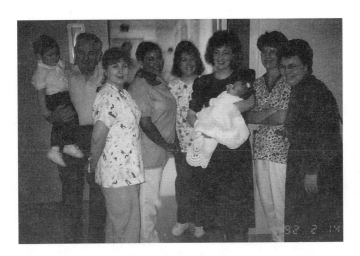

Farewells from the nursing staff.

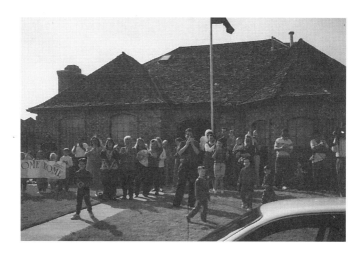

Valentine's Day — Heidi's first view of home.

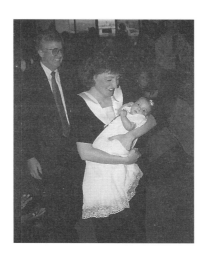

Baby dedication, two weeks after arriving home.

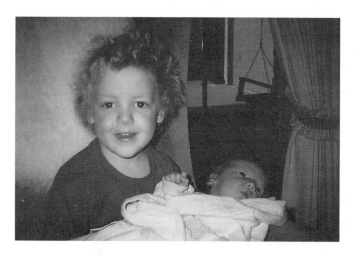

April 1996 — A sleepy Heidi welcomes her new brother.

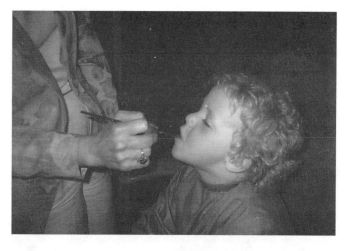

June 1996 — Her favorite thing about television taping?
"Lick stick" and makeup!

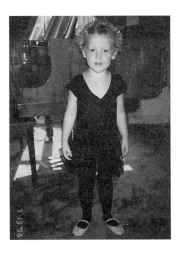

July 1996 — First day of ballet.

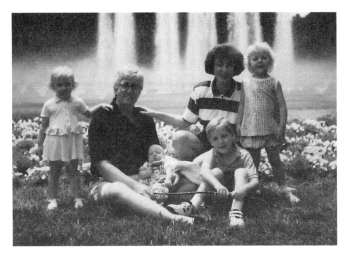

Summer 1996 — Our family today.

Chapter Ten

I Hate Sundays!

The next afternoon, the hospital chaplain stopped by to see us. Chaplain Martin was in his late fifties, a white-haired gentle, gracious man. We had met him at the beginning of Heidi's hospital stay. After realizing the extent of our support group and the involvement of our own spiritual community in the situation, he had not visited her bedside but had encouraged us to call him should we need his assistance. We frequently passed him in the hallways and had chatted briefly on several occasions.

So we found it interesting that he was making his fourth visit to Heidi's bedside in the past six days. Although kind and gentle, it was obvious to us that we frustrated his plan for each of those visits. That's when we realized he had been brought in as a participant in the Reality Campaign. His report for Heidi's chart made it even clearer:

I saw the family on the 18th of December and subsequently on the 20th, the 21st and the 23rd. Offered support to the family, really largely at the urging of the attending physician. Tried to get the family to talk about the *real* circumstance with this patient. This, they were unwilling to do and expressed that unwillingness, saying they really didn't want to talk about anything that was negative in front of the baby. That is verbatim. So, I continued to offer support to them and to the grandparents and encouraged them, of course, to follow their own spiritual support community in any way they chose to. I saw them repeatedly but the situation really did not change.

Even the hospital chaplain didn't know what to do with us! With each passing day we were more aware that the medical community was not going to understand us. They didn't have to. The important thing was that we were all working together toward Heidi's healing. Our job was to continue to stand in faith and fight the battle for her complete healing. And the medical staff was doing a superb job of taking care of their part. Many of the staff were also becoming dear friends with the grandparents and with us.

As we reflected over the previous day when Heidi had come off the respirator, we both voiced what we had thought several times over the past weeks.

"Vickie, have you noticed that every Sunday, the battle has gotten worse?" Chuck asked me.

"Yes. I didn't want to admit it. But yesterday left no doubt in my mind," I answered.

"And during the morning hours when so many church bodies are praying together for her—those seem to be the toughest," he added.

"I never thought I'd say this, Chuck. But I'm starting to dread Sundays!"

The weeks were filled with plenty of skirmishes with the enemy, but Sundays were World War III! The battle was especially intense then. No doubt about it. We had both come to view the arrival of each Sunday with trepidation. We were usually able to attend the worship service at our church. The opportunity to corporately praise God for what He was doing in our lives was like feasting at a banquet table. And the tremendous love and support from the people was our dessert. But when we left that service, we went from the banquet table to the battle trenches.

On the first Sunday of Heidi's life, the doctors had been forced to start prostaglandin, the emergency heart medicine, to buy a few weeks' time while she hopefully improved. Remember, they had hoped they wouldn't have to use this medication because of the bad side effects. That had been a frightening day as we watched her condition careen downhill.

Sunday number two, December 1, was the "best of the worst" although there were repeated problems with IV lines closing down.

On her third Sunday, we fought spiritual warfare with the spirit of death. It was a day of intense battle. God won, Satan lost, but we were weary, wounded warriors.

And on Sunday number four she went into congestive heart failure while the heart ductus closed. Her oxygen saturation levels dipped lower and lower as her heart struggled to carry the load.

We had just survived the Sunday of December 22—our seventeen-hour day when Heidi fought her way off the respirator. We were grateful to be off the respirator, but it had been a long bloody battle.

I think even the Gallup Polls would call this a definite trend! But what were we to do? Sunday was going to continue to come once every seven days. And we certainly weren't going to ask people to stop praying. But each week by late Saturday night, we found ourselves bracing for the onslaught of the enemy.

Meanwhile, this was the week of Christmas. How relieved I was that all of my Christmas shopping and gift wrapping had been completed before Heidi's birth. That pregnancy nesting instinct can pay great dividends!

My Scrooge tendencies had thankfully disappeared. We both wanted to make Christmas Day a special time for Sterling. Thanks to his three grandparents, he had been able to enjoy the thousands of lights in our subdivision on early evening walks or drives.

Grandma Watson went home to Ohio for several days that week to celebrate with the rest of the Watson family in Tipp City.

Early Christmas morning, Chuck and I opened gifts with Sterling around our tree. It was a precious time because he was able to respond so much more this year as an almost-two-year-old.

Yet it was difficult to keep pushing aside the mental images I had while wrapping those gifts six weeks earlier. A fire glowing in the fireplace, Christmas tree lights twinkling, carols playing in the background, and new baby Watson nestled in an infant seat beside the brick hearth as we opened presents. No, the season had been vastly different, and yet, there was so much to be grateful for—"new baby Watson" was alive and off the respirator.

We joined Mother and Dad mid-morning at Bryan's and Rose Annette's house, just eight minutes away in Hurst, to exchange gifts and enjoy Christmas dinner. Ed was at the hospital with Heidi until noon so we could have this family time together. People like Ed had continued to give sacrificially of their time even during the busy holiday season.

My sister's house had always been a place where I could let down and relax. As I settled into the comfortable recliner in Rose Annette's family room, I realized that this was the first time for us to all be together since Mother's and Dad's arrival six and one-half weeks earlier. All together except for Heidi. Sterling enjoyed Jeremy and Jessica as usual. And with a two-, six-, and eight-year-old present, there was plenty of excitement and laughter with the unwrapping of gifts. It was good to be brought back into a slice of "normal life."

We adults were mellower than usual—partially from physical weariness. Mother had stayed all night at the hospital with Heidi. She gave her a doll and proudly reported that they had played dolls during the night!

She had picked up Daddy at our house at seven that morning, and they had come to watch Jeremy and Jessica when they awakened to their gifts. So with zero sleep, she was pushing her limits. The long haul was taking its toll on all of us.

Yet we were able to enjoy this special time together and share our gratitude for what God was doing in our family's life. The trappings and commercialism of Christmas were not the least bit seductive that year. And the real meaning—God's gift of His Son Jesus—was more precious than ever.

We relaxed so much that the time slipped away. Before we knew it, we needed to leave for the hospital to relieve Ed so he could enjoy the rest of the day with his family. Rose Annette, with the help of her family, had prepared a feast—turkey, dressing, green beans, mashed potatoes with gravy, cranberry sauce, squash casserole, sweet potato casserole, homemade rolls, fruit salad, and pecan pie. Because it was so late, Chuck and I ate our Christmas dinner on paper plates in the van while driving to the hospital. Different yet delicious!

We left Sterling to enjoy the rest of the day with the family. Bryan and Rose Annette would spend that night with Heidi.

Christmas Day in the NICU. It was a quiet peaceful afternoon. Not many people in the unit. The only unusual thing was the privacy screen which they placed around one of the beds shortly after we arrived. We held Heidi and rocked her for most of the afternoon. We had made pictures with her on Christmas Eve. I couldn't wait to see them because Heidi looked so much better to me.

When Chuck showed me the prints of those photos the next week, I was astounded. There was a beaming mother with a frighteningly blue child. I couldn't believe how dark her coloring was from the lack of oxygen. It was the first time I realized that I was blocking out some things—my method of coping. And there were other things that God was protecting me from seeing. He was keeping my focus on Him and what He said about Heidi. Later we were all amazed at the details which Chuck, Mother, or Rose Annette would relate for which I had no memory. I had been there physically, but sometimes God and sometimes I had not allowed them to compute emotionally.

Mid-afternoon on Christmas Day, I mentioned the privacy screen around the one baby's bed to Chuck. He nodded without comment. In the waiting room during the shift change that night, he explained. "Vickie, that baby died right after we arrived. I'm sorry. I thought you knew what was happening."

Ohhh! The reality of where we were stung! This was the Neonatal Intensive Care Unit. All of these babies were in critical condition. Some would not make it. That could have been Heidi. She had been so close so many times. And one of her roommates had died on Christmas afternoon. No, this wasn't where we would have chosen to spend Christmas. And yet we were grateful in another sense to still be there. Our baby was alive. *Thank you, God.*

Driving home in the van that evening, much earlier than usual, we listened to the news on the radio. Small doses of normalcy were good for us that day. In four and one-half weeks I had been nowhere except home, hospital, church, and the doctor's office. I had not cooked a meal, washed a load of laundry, cleaned my house, or shopped for groceries. Our needs had been abundantly supplied. And I had been enabled to focus on caring for Sterling and Heidi. God had been very gracious to us in every way.

We were almost home when we heard the radio announcer refer to that week's top news story—the bringing down of the Berlin Wall. We looked at each other incredulously.

"Did he say that the Berlin Wall came down?" I was not sure I had heard correctly.

"That's what he said! I can't believe it! And we haven't heard a thing about it. Talk about being out of touch with what's going on in the world! I wonder what else has happened during the last month. If the Berlin Wall could come down without our hearing a peep about it, there's no telling what else we've missed!" Chuck replied.

We had to laugh. The focus of our lives had changed so much. And yet the focus was where it was supposed to be for this season. Whatever it took, our number one priority was the battle for Heidi's life.

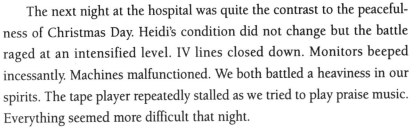

The next night at the hospital was quite the contrast to the peacefulness of Christmas Day. Heidi's condition did not change but the battle raged at an intensified level. IV lines closed down. Monitors beeped incessantly. Machines malfunctioned. We both battled a heaviness in our spirits. The tape player repeatedly stalled as we tried to play praise music. Everything seemed more difficult that night.

The nurse walked over at one point and asked, "Do you feel this? There's some kind of magnetic field causing the machinery to malfunction. We've had this happen a few times before. But this time I can actually feel it in the air. Do you?"

"Oh, yes," we assured her. "We are very aware of it."

It had been going on for three hours. Pete the respiratory therapist was doing Heidi's breathing treatment when Pastor Jim arrived. The breathing treatments consisted of a medicated mist which she would breathe for ten minutes, followed by a "pounding" on her chest and back to loosen the mucous in her lungs. It sounded and looked painful although it was not. It ended with a suction tube being placed down each nostril to suction out the loosened mucous. Although very effective, that part was painful.

When Pete started the "pounding" the pastor asked him several questions. The first time observing this treatment was usually difficult for anyone. Although Pete had done her breathing treatment many times, and we had gotten to know him well, tonight seemed harder for some reason. Heidi was crying and kept looking at me with her big eyes, begging for intervention. The tears silently rolled down my cheeks as I watched, unable to do anything about her crying. We had to keep her lungs as clear as possible. I just didn't know why everything seemed so much harder on this night.

After explaining what he was doing, Pete started asking the pastor questions. "Are you a minister?"

"Yes, I am," he replied.

"What kind of minister?" asked Pete.

"I'm a Protestant minister."

"Well, I'm a minister too," Pete replied. We all looked up with surprise. Chuck and I had enjoyed many conversations with Pete, but he had never mentioned this.

"What kind of minister are you, Pete?" questioned Jim.

"I'm a Hindu priest," he replied.

"Umph," was the only sound from Pastor Jim.

The three of us felt like we had been punched in the stomach. The heaviness descended even further. There was no more conversation. The tears flowed faster down my cheeks as I held onto Heidi's hand.

God, where are you? Where are your warring angels? It's time to show up! The nurses even sense the battle. And a Hindu priest is pounding on my daughter!

As soon as the breathing treatment ended, the three of us started praying softly with fervor. Our mothers were there to relieve us, but we knew we could not leave Heidi until there was a change. There were fiery darts flying everywhere.

When I walked Pastor Jim to the waiting room, I realized just how intense the battle was. I could hardly walk because of the heaviness. It felt as if someone was pressing downward on my shoulders with his full weight.

Returning to Heidi's bedside, I found Chuck staring out the window at her side. The hour was late. The courtyard below was deserted. The sky was filled with twinkling stars.

His face was white as he turned to look at me. "I just saw it, Vickie. I literally saw the battle! The sky right outside the window was filled with angels and demons in intense conflict. The battle was over Heidi's life—a real war within a cloud outside her window. A war between light and darkness, good and evil, life and death! Swords were flying everywhere. It was just like in Frank Peretti's book, *This Present Darkness*."

I recalled the vivid word pictures painted in Peretti's book of the spiritual battle between the powers of good and evil. Although I had not seen it with my eyes, it certainly was what the night had felt like. Intense warfare. I wasn't about to leave my baby in the midst of this—no matter how late the hour.

"But it's okay to leave Heidi now," he continued as if reading my thoughts. "God won. The battle is over for the night."

We realized then that no alarms had buzzed for the past ten minutes. Calmness had returned. We now refer to that night as our "This Present Darkness Night."

The Sunday following Christmas brought good news. Heidi came off of the CPAP. She was now breathing totally on her own! We raced to her bedside that afternoon to see her. Only one tube left on her face—a feeding tube down her mouth and into her stomach. Her heart was still too weak to take on the task of a bottle. She would have used more calories to drink the milk than she could have gotten from the milk itself. But she looked beautiful! This was the closest I had come to seeing her entire face since her birth. Only two strips of tape and one small tube left! She still had the surgical IV line in her chest and the heart monitor, but we were getting there! And it was Sunday!

That afternoon Chuck and I relaxed as we enjoyed a quiet afternoon with Heidi and nurse Sarah. I rocked Heidi for a long time while we chatted.

"It's Sunday. No bombs," I whispered to Chuck.

"I know. Maybe the Sunday curse is broken. I'm holding my breath until the day is over," he replied. "But she is off the CPAP. And it was much easier than coming off the respirator."

We were both glad to see the CPAP tube gone. The irritation of a tube down her nasal passage had caused a constant flow of thick mucous. You could hear her breathing across the room. The nurse had mentioned that some babies fight the CPAP tube even more than the respirator. It had been an uncomfortable week for Heidi, so we were grateful to see the exit of another tube.

When he arrived on the unit, Dr. Smith pulled up a chair and joined us. He seemed to enjoy the relaxed atmosphere for a change also. After visiting about the holidays for a few minutes, he brought us up to date on Heidi's condition.

"Well, as you can see, she is off the CPAP. I'm really pleased at how she has done in the five hours since we took it off. We did a sonogram this morning of the heart and lung areas. There is good news and bad news."

No! Sundays were going to be different now. No more bad news on Sunday. I stopped rocking. We both waited motionless.

"The good news is that her heart is continuing to get smaller. We want to hold off on the transplant option at this point. So we won't be sending her to Dallas next week. She'll stay here for now."

It was wonderful news! That's what we had wanted to hear. But what was the bad news? We found ourselves bracing for the lowering of the boom.

Dr. Smith continued. "Dr. Dambro had requested the sonogram of the lung area because Heidi's breathing should have improved more since coming off the respirator. All this week, she has felt as if there must be another contributing factor to the problems with breathing. When we did the sonogram this morning, we discovered that her right diaphragm is paralyzed."

"How did that happen?" Chuck asked.

"Well, there are several possibilities. And we'll never know which is accurate. It could have been that way at birth, and we would not have known because she went on the respirator immediately. It would not show up as long as she was on the respirator. It could have been damaged when inserting the respirator tube. You know it's been in and out several times, and some of those times were emergency situations when we were putting it back in."

"So what does this mean?" Chuck voiced the question in both our minds. "What do we do to fix it?"

"There is really nothing we can do to fix it. It makes breathing more difficult for her, and she doesn't need to have anything else compromising her breathing. She needs everything possible going for her at this point, as you well know. There are instances where diaphragms start working on their own. But that usually happens fairly quickly. She has been off the respirator for a week now. The longer it stays paralyzed, the less likely that it will ever work," he concluded.

"Well," I said quietly starting to rock again and snuggling Heidi closer, "we've seen heart medications go. We've seen the respirator go. We've seen a heart decrease in size. We'll just add that to our list. Next we'll do a right diaphragm."

Nurse Sarah looked down at Heidi and then at Dr. Smith. "It *is* that time of year, you know. Christmas. Babies. Miracles."

"Well, yeah. Okay. We'll see what happens," was his reply.

Although it certainly wasn't encouraging news, it didn't blow us away. We added it to the prayer list, right under "functioning tricuspid valve." Satan was not going to steal our victory this Sunday. Heidi was breathing on room air, and we were grateful. God could handle a diaphragm that needed to start moving.

We had one difficult task ahead of us that evening. On Friday night, another of Heidi's roommates had died. But this time it was closer. It was Tara. Each of us had gotten close to her parents and grandmother. And God had allowed us to minister to them through prayer and conversations. I didn't think Tara would die. I thought she was going to make it. We were standing in prayer and faith, believing for her healing and her parents' salvation. So this one hit hard.

After we left the hospital that night, Chuck and I visited with Scott and Raina at the funeral home. The tiny casket. Tara's little body which I had prayed over each time I walked by her bed on the way to Heidi's. It was a painful reminder of how close Heidi had been to death so many times over the past five and one-half weeks. This could have been us.

We then understood why the nurses had seemed emotionally distant during Heidi's lowest times. I recalled a recent conversation I had overheard between a respiratory therapist and one of the nurses. The therapist was telling the nurse about a new baby brought in that morning by helicopter. The baby was in serious condition. But what had stuck with me was her final comment, "And you don't want to meet the family." At the time it seemed like a cruel remark. Several hours later I heard the two talking again about the same baby. The nurse said, "You were right about the family. They are precious. This is going to be a hard one." Then I understood. The medical staff paid a high emotional price for getting close to these families. It was a tightrope balancing act to give loving care and yet keep emotional equilibrium. And they dealt with this daily.

As we left the funeral home, we realized we could not handle the funeral the next day. Grandpa Ed went to represent our family and minister to Scott and Raina.

———————— ➤ ————————

The next week brought the beginning of 1992 and a special beginning for Heidi. At 6:00 a.m. on New Year's Day, Mother, Sue (a friend who along with her husband Carl had stayed all night), and Nurse Chris moved Heidi across the hall from Side A (Critical Care) to Side B (Intermediate Care) of the NICU. We had finally made it to Side B! It was still Intensive Care, but these babies were off respirators. There was the sound of crying. It was beautiful!

Forty days and forty nights on Side A. I felt as if we had lived through the flood, and the dove had just returned to our ark with an olive branch for Noah. What a wonderful way to start the new year!

Within twenty-four hours, Heidi had a fever and major congestion. Her breathing was labored. And her constant coughing was taxing on her heart. Within a matter of hours, she didn't even have the strength to cough. It was pitiful.

Dr. Smith called us at home to explain. "Our concern is that this may be RSV—respiratory synctial virus. To you or me that's usually manifested as a cold. To babies with heart and lung problems, it can be deadly. It is the most contagious virus we deal with. We're testing her for it and will have tentative results tomorrow. But we won't have final results back until next week. Meanwhile if anyone in your family has a cold, tell them to stay away from the hospital."

I had thought nothing of the minor cold I had been nursing for several days. But now it meant I couldn't see Heidi. I was tested for RSV in the emergency room of our local hospital that afternoon. By the following afternoon (Friday), Heidi's symptoms had worsened, and they moved her into an isolation room off of Side A.

The doctor recorded the developments on Heidi's chart:

> Mother ELISA [test] positive for RSV. Baby has increased cough but stable. Baby's ELISA negative for RSV. Since RSV would be devastating and possibly fatal to this child, and Ribovirin aerosol relatively benign treatment, we will treat with Ribovirin and repeat the culture [test]. Will not allow mother to visit until she is ELISA negative.

So they began treating Heidi for RSV with a medicated mist in a tent. Although her initial test showed that she did not have the virus, she continued to have every symptom of it. The final test results would take three days. And they could not wait for three more days to start the treatment. It would be too late then if she did have it. Dr. Dambro had also noted on her chart—*Patient at very high risk if she gets this infection.*

In the back of my mind was the nagging thought—if she gets it, she got it from me. I had snuggled her in my arms for hours over the past few days. There was no doubt for the medical staff. They had battled this virus once before in the NICU. It was almost impossible to contain an outbreak because it was so contagious. And some babies didn't survive it. There was no way I could have held Heidi with a cold—that turned out to be RSV—and not transmitted the virus to her. They were also concerned as to how many other babies could have already been infected by passing it through Heidi's nurses.

Nurses and supplies were labeled either "clean" or "dirty." Any nurse who had taken care of Heidi in the last two days was not allowed on the floor of the unit. They could only care for Heidi in the isolation room. They roped off one entrance and scrubbing area of the NICU for those entering Heidi's room. All others entered the unit by a separate entrance.

That Friday and Saturday, I worked at putting my energy into something positive. I couldn't be with Heidi, but there were other things that could be done. I answered the phones to give the volunteers a break. After a day and a half of that—we were still receiving an average of thirty calls a day for updates on Heidi—I understood why God had provided other people to give the updates on her condition and keep the prayer chain advised. The medical facts had to be stated so that people would know how to pray. And yet by the time I had stated those facts thirty times, my focus was far from what God had told me about Heidi. It would have been impossible for me to have done this over the past weeks while still holding on to any remnant of faith for Heidi's healing. God knew that, and He had graciously provided.

Saturday afternoon I felt that my time and energy were to go toward preparing for Heidi's homecoming. Our parents and many volunteers had done a masterful job of running the household. But there was always plenty of work to be done. Chuck's mother tackled the stack of ironing. And mother and I worked on the house—putting things away, organizing the boxes of dishes to be returned, and cleaning. Mother and I work well together because we both appreciate order. And doing the housework felt good. It was another slice of normal life.

I even ran to the grocery store to get milk for Sterling. Venturing back into the mechanics of living gave me new hope that Heidi would be coming home soon and doing those things with us. As I waited in the check-out line at Kroger, my eyes swept over the people standing in line. Immediately to my left was one of the special carts that has an infant carrier welded onto it. *Oh, no!* My mind went into instant panic. There was probably a baby there. I wasn't ready for this. Another newborn out and about, enjoying life. What if I did something drastic? I could see myself going over to a startled new mother and saying—"Do you know how blessed you are to have your baby here with you? Do you understand what a gift the health of this child is? Do you have any idea what it means to leave your baby every day? To have a six and one-half week old who has never left the hospital? To be waiting for the day when you can see what your child's face looks like without strips of tape covering portions of it? Do you know what a miracle it is that your baby is lying there smiling at you? **Do you know?**"

I quickly moved to a check-out line several aisles over. *Get a grip on yourself, Vickie. This is real life, and you're going to have to face it sooner or later.*

I realized that I had been mercifully sheltered from many painful situations since Heidi's birth. I never knew how I would respond emotionally to a situation. Our first Sunday back at church after Heidi's birth (December 1), we had unknowingly sat down behind a couple whose baby girl was born six days after Heidi. There she lay nestled in the infant carrier right in front of our eyes. Lynn and Kim were apologetic.

"Oh, no," we responded. "It's okay. It's good to see a healthy newborn. It's right that she is here with you. We've seen so many critically ill babies in the last ten days that we've forgotten what it's supposed to be like. This is a good reminder for us. We're grateful that she's healthy. We don't want anyone else to ever have to go through this."

So the emotional intensity of the grocery store episode surprised me. I never knew from one minute to the next what I would be able to handle. I was on an emotional roller coaster.

The next morning, January 5, Chuck, Sterling, our mothers, and I attended church together. Dad was at the hospital with Heidi. Last Sunday had been so much better that we had found ourselves hopeful going into this day. It had been the beginning of a new kind of Sunday.

Heidi was still in isolation and obviously battling all of the symptoms of RSV, but the doctors were hopeful that they had caught it soon enough. Chuck and our parents had explained to me how difficult it was for her to breathe. They were suctioning massive amounts of mucous from her breathing passages every hour. But we all knew that Heidi was a fighter.

The praise in the beginning moments of the church service ministered deeply to us. We were once again able to refill our near empty tanks. There was a powerful lengthy time of prayer for Heidi and the RSV. We felt the presence of God as many surrounded us at the altar. We were boosted by the faithful and intense intercession of our church family on our behalf.

As we returned to our seats, Chuck hugged me close and said, "It's going to be okay. She's going to make it through RSV too."

"Yes, she is. Isn't God good, honey?"

We had been in our seats less than three minutes when an usher tapped Chuck on the shoulder. "The hospital is on the telephone. It's an emergency. They need to talk to both of you," he whispered.

I couldn't believe it. *No, there must be a mistake. We were through with this kind of Sunday. What could have happened that they would call us at church?* A team of intercessors followed us to the phones. I was in the kitchen on one extension and Chuck was through the door in the larger meeting room using a telephone there. "This is Chuck Watson."

"Mr. and Mrs. Watson, are you both there?" Dr. Juliao responded immediately to Chuck's tense voice.

"Yes, we're both here," Chuck replied. "What's happened?"

"We just had to put Heidi back on the respirator. I am so sorry. Her coughing spells have lasted two to three minutes. And the thick secretions finally blocked her airways totally. We thought we were going to lose her for a little while. We had no choice but to put her back on the respirator. She wasn't breathing. I am so very sorry."

Every doctor had shared in our elation when Heidi had come off the respirator, so they knew this was a painful step backward for us. But the bigger picture was that she had stopped breathing. Dr. Juliao had recorded: *cyanosis . . . no air exchange . . . prolonged expiratory phase.* There had been a painfully long time when she wasn't breathing.

"Mr. and Mrs. Watson, you need to come down here right away. We have sedated her with morphine, but if this same thing happens on the respirator, there are no options left. We're using every measure to thin the secretions, but it hasn't been enough. That's why this virus can be deadly for children like Heidi."

"But what about my wife, Dr. Juliao? They said she can't come into the hospital until she tests negative for RSV," Chuck reminded him.

"Well, we don't have a choice right now. We have to make a way for you to see her. She's in serious shape. We'll work it out somehow. Come to the side entrance, and we'll have a nurse meet you there with sterile gown, mask, and gloves. You'll need to put them on before entering the hospital. And don't sit down in the waiting room or use the telephone. Basically you're not to touch anything between the entrance and Heidi's bedside," Dr. Juliao concluded.

I had listened and cried through the entire conversation. When we hung up, Chuck called the NICU waiting room knowing that Dad would be there until they allowed him back in the room. I couldn't even talk for crying. As Chuck asked him about it, Dad's tearful response painted a frightening picture. "It was really rough. She stopped breathing. It was a long time." He tearfully repeated those words to each of Chuck's questions. It had been traumatic for him as well.

People spontaneously gathered around us in the meeting room to pray before we left. It was a major blow to all of us. Chuck was crying and yet skillfully handling the necessary arrangements. Our mothers would stay at church and take Sterling home for the afternoon. Someone else was driving Chuck and me to the hospital. I felt as if I was in a fog watching all of this happening. And it was so cold in there. Someone had gotten our coats out of the service, and I was wrapped up, but I could not get warm.

As we started down the hallway, I mumbled something to Chuck about how cold it was. He put me in the car and ran back inside, returning a minute later with Judy, a friend who is a nurse. She had decided to go with us. The lady driving us "happened" to have a quilt in her trunk. "I've been forgetting to put that away, and now I know why. You needed it today," she smiled as she handed it to Chuck. I laid my head on his lap in the backseat, shaking uncontrollably beneath my heavy coat and the quilt. My body had reached its emotional limit. I didn't realize until several days later that I was in shock. That's why Chuck had asked Judy to go with us. To this day, I don't remember the drive to the hospital or who drove us or our arrival there. I do remember walking through the waiting room and being puzzled as to how Rich and Sharon knew to be there. These friends were spiritual warriors who attended another church. I later learned that in the middle of their worship service that morning, Sharon had leaned over to Rich and said, "We're to pray for Heidi. Something's going on." The heaviness in her spirit did not lift by the end of the service, and they headed straight to the hospital, arriving only minutes before us. Judy brought them up to date as we headed to Heidi's bedside.

Entering the unit, we saw Dr. Lai. "I am so sorry," he said. "I think all of the doctors on the case have seen this coming for about twenty-four hours. And none of us wanted to be the one to put Heidi back on the respirator. We took it as far as we could."

"We're not questioning your decision. Dr. Juliao told us on the phone that she would have died had he not put her back on. We understand. It's just not what any of us wanted to happen," Chuck said.

"Well, we just all feel so badly." Dr. Lai headed across the NICU.

I remember that it seemed to take forever to scrub in and change gown, mask, and gloves even though I had just put them on at the entrance. I was still in a fog. My only thought was that I didn't want to see that respirator tube again—not on my Heidi.

The area where we scrubbed, and the closet sized enclosure (used for passing supplies) that led into Heidi's isolation room, were roped off. It reminded me of a crime scene. It was my first time in the tiny isolation room where she had been for the past three days. Dad, Chuck, the nurse, and I totally filled the remaining floor space. As we walked in, Dad hugged me, still wiping tears from his eyes as he said, "She's had a rough morning, Vic." For Dad to say that, I knew it had been a frighteningly close call.

Heidi's nurse greeted us with tears in her eyes, "I'm so sorry." She couldn't say more.

I searched for Heidi amidst the machinery. There was the large tent delivering the RSV medication. The respirator tubes snaked their way across the bed. The IVs. Morphine. And there in the middle was tiny, motionless Heidi. I felt as if we had just gone backward by a mile. Could we recover from this one? She looked lifeless. The one sign of life was the horrible sound of congestion with each mechanical breath from the respirator.

Dr. Juliao came in, apologizing again for her being back on the respirator. "We need to discuss the isolation issue. Your family should not eat here at the hospital, or use the waiting room. You could pass this to another family who would then take it to their sick child. We would have an epidemic on our hands. We cannot risk that."

"What about pumping my breast milk?" I knew that would be a necessity within a couple of hours.

"Oh, no, you'll have to use your own pump. And you can't go in that room because other mothers could pick up germs and spread them to the babies," he explained.

Meekly I asked, "What about using the restroom?"

"No, I—well I guess we don't have a choice. You have to be able to do that. But please don't touch anything with your bare hands. Your family along with these nurses and everything in this room including me is considered dirty," Dr. Juliao said.

I felt like Hester in *The Scarlet Letter* and wondered if the next step would be to embroider "RSV" in red letters on the bodice of the sterile hospital gowns I would wear. Of course none of this was as important as Heidi's condition. But we knew it was another weapon in Satan's arsenal. Kick them while they're down. Hit them with extra emotional strain at their weak moment. Just keep hurling things at them one right after the other. They don't even all have to be biggies. The biggie is taken care of. Heidi is on the brink of life and death again. But now make it harder for them to function here. Not able to eat on the premises. Not able to relax in the waiting room. That will also take care of the ministry that's been going on with other NICU families. Not able to use the breast pump facilities. That pump at home weighs about fifty pounds. That'll be a real pain to carry back and forth. And make Vickie feel guilty for causing all of this. She's close to her limit. It won't take much for her to forget she ever heard the song, "You Are A Masterpiece."

The rest of the day? Heidi's heart rate kept climbing to the 200 range so they discussed putting her on a paralyzing drug to keep her from burning so many calories. The IV in her foot collapsed so they had to put a new one in her head. They took her off of breast milk through the stomach tube because she was vomiting. She required continual morphine to keep her from fighting the tube.

The new isolation requirements made the night shift especially difficult for our mothers. The bathroom was the only place they could go for a break. There was no place they could lie down or even sit except for the stool at Heidi's bedside. The hospital was in a dangerous section of Fort Worth so it was too risky to go to the car during the night for a quick nap.

It was a long day and night. What did I learn from Sunday, January 5, 1992?

I hate Sundays! I hate them! I hate them! I hate them!

Chapter Eleven

My "Job" Day

"Be ruthless with yourself if you are given to talking about the experiences you have had. Faith that is sure of itself is not faith; faith that is sure of God is the only faith there is." [9]

I awoke that Monday morning to an emotional weariness like I had not yet known. Our bedroom seemed darker than usual for eight o'clock. The late night hospital visits had pushed our bedtime to one-thirty or two a.m., so our body clocks had started alarming around eight o'clock most mornings. Although the elegant drapes, along with the mini blinds and sheers, kept out most of the light, I could still tell it was an overcast, gray, January day—just the way I felt.

As I looked around our bedroom, the memories of the past six and one-half weeks awakened for yet another painful day. At the foot of our bed sat the small white cradle—the same pink sheet, Sterling's fluffy lamb in the corner, Grandma's afghan still folded neatly across the bottom, and no baby. Nothing had changed since November. Three large windows formed an alcove which looked out onto the quiet residential street. In front of the window sat the blue rocking recliner—my thirty-seventh birthday gift from Chuck last August. It's a sign of age when you request a recliner for your birthday! The motionless recliner had not yet rocked a mother and newborn. At that moment, I could not imagine ever complaining about four a.m. feedings again.

The changing table, in front of the window, was readied for action. The top shelf with padded cushion awaited a baby with a dirty diaper. Two lower shelves were laden with diapers, gowns, outfits, booties, and receiving blankets all in perfect stacks. Those stacks should have been messed up by now—the way they get when you're holding a squirming baby lying on the top shelf with one hand while you search for a clean gown with the other hand and keep the baby's feet out of a smelly mess with another hand. Yes, mothers do have three hands!

On the wall, hanging from a wooden curio shelf, were Heidi's long white christening gown and cap. I had decided weeks ago not to change the miniature red rose and ribbon on the gown to pink. The red had become a symbolic reminder of Jesus' blood every time I had looked at it. Until this morning.

The view from my bed had given me hope many times over the past weeks. But the word "hope" had vanished from my emotional vocabulary that day. I pulled the pale pink down comforter tighter around my shoulders, but that did not phase the cold within. As I rolled over in our queen size bed, realizing that my husband Chuck was already awake, I snuggled into his warm embrace seeking comfort for the ache that wouldn't go away. We lay there silently for a few minutes holding each other.

No, it wasn't a bad dream. It was January 6, 1992. Heidi was forty-seven days old today and continued to fight for life in the Neonatal Intensive Care Unit at Cook Children's Medical Center. Yes, before her birth, God had told me that she was fearfully and wonderfully made and that she would grow up and her life would be a miracle. But yes, her heart had stopped beating yesterday. She had stopped breathing. And yes, she had gone back on the respirator for the third time. It had been a Sunday. What else did I expect?

This was not one of my finest "spiritual" moments. In fact it was my lowest. I poured out the dredges of my emotional lake to Chuck as we lay in bed that dreary winter morning.

"I don't know how much more I can take. I can't watch my baby suffer any more. I'm tired of people saying what a difference it has made in their lives. My baby suffers so they can get straightened out spiritually?

No deal!

"I feel like Job, sitting in the dirt with a broken piece of pottery, scraping my boils. (The Bible records the story of Job, a godly man, who lost family, possessions and health.) I don't know what it is that God expects of us, but this is too much. We're only human. I'm ready to say, 'Either heal her or take her.'

"We've been taught to stand firmly on what He tells us about a situation. And He has told me clearly about Heidi. But it's been forty-seven days and *nothing* matches up. I have stood on His Word . . . I have spoken His Word . . . I have planned our future based on His Word . . . yet what I see with my eyes continues to go in the opposite direction from what He has said.

"What am I supposed to do with what I feel? He says to stand on His Word, and yet He gave me emotions. What do I do with them?"

My dear husband, who can in seconds go from a sound sleep to an animated telephone conversation, held me in his arms silently. I slowly realized that this was one of those rare times when Chuck and I hit bottom together. I was farther down in the hole than he, but not by much. So he wasn't able to pull me out. We were there together.

After several minutes of weary silence, he tenderly replied, "I don't know, honey. I don't understand either. But what are our choices? We both know we want to see her healed. I hurt as badly for you, watching you go through this, as I do for Heidi. I just want to fix it for both of you—for all of us. But I don't know what else to do. We've got to keep taking one step at a time each day. We can't give up on her."

Then he telephoned Mike and Adrienne, faithful friends only blocks away who had listened many times before. They arrived within minutes and entered with their usual bedroom greeting over the last weeks— "Open these blinds and get some light in here. Get out of bed and get dressed. That alone will do wonders for your spirits." But no bright sunshine flooded the room or my spirit that morning as they raised the blinds and pulled back the sheers. It was overcast without and within. The four of us sat on our bed, Mike and Adrienne dressed for their day as airline pilot and mother of five, Chuck in his navy and white Japanese robe, and me in my soft warm forest green robe. True friends know what you look like in your robe and with the scant remains of yesterday morning's make-up.

As I repeated my thoughts to them, Adrienne's first response was, "I'm certainly not going to be one of Job's friends. I don't have anything to tell you!" (God told Eliphaz, one of Job's friends, "My wrath is kindled against thee, and against thy two friends: for ye have not spoken of Me the thing that is right, as My servant Job hath." Job 42:7, KJV) Adrienne's gift of humor in the middle of the crisis was right on target as usual.

As we knelt beside the bed to pray, I reiterated to Mike and Adrienne, "I'm ready to say to God, 'Either heal her or take her.'"

"Then, say it! God can handle that," encouraged Adrienne.

"But I can't bring myself to say those words to Him, knowing what God really wants for her—that she will grow up and her life will be a miracle. I've got to know where my limits are with God. What can I say to Him without crossing an invisible boundary as His child? How angry will He allow me to be with Him?"

As they prayed for us—since neither of us had any praying left within—the intensity of my emotions subsided. But I still didn't have my answer. How angry *would* God allow me to be with Him?

Mike, exhibiting his military training, firmly announced, "We are going out for breakfast. You have been living at the hospital and this house for forty-seven days, and you've got to take a break. You have fifteen minutes to be dressed. And we won't take no for an answer."

Twenty minutes later, we headed for the back door. Before leaving the house, we stopped by the kitchen table to read the grandmothers' notes from their night at the hospital. They usually returned home each morning just as Grandpa Boone was leaving for his daytime shift. Months later my parents shared with me their ritual of good-morning/good-night kisses in our driveway at six-thirty a.m. each morning. It had not dawned on me that they did not get to sleep together during those long months of vigil at the hospital.

This morning's notes revealed that Heidi had a restless night—fever of 101 degrees, did a blood culture, more vomiting, morphine at 4:20 a.m., still in isolation. But this morning I didn't expect any positive news from the night.

Breakfast at IHOP provided a welcome relief. The world had actually continued on during those forty-seven days. People were going to work, going out to eat, shopping, traveling. Life had moved on even though we had not. As we sat in the blue vinyl booth across from Mike and Adrienne, the waitress took our orders for Harvest Grain and Nut pancakes. The decision between maple and boysenberry syrup seemed so easy after the surgery and transplant decisions of the previous month. Our waitress provided comic relief as she served us. Through her work, she brought joy to others in spite of a mental handicap. Adrienne and I found ourselves laughing with her each time she came to our table. It was good to know that I could still laugh. However, the heaviness did not lift for Chuck during breakfast.

Arriving back home, we slipped quietly in the front door and on into our bedroom, realizing that Sterling was playing contentedly in the family room at the back of the house with Mary, a precious grandmother from our church family. Our stomachs felt better, full of pancakes, eggs, and bacon. The glimpse of ongoing life had been helpful for me. Chuck had those glimpses each time he went to his office so it had not seemed unusual to him. But our return home brought back for me the heaviness and the reminder of what our life consisted of at this time.

Chuck headed to his office at American Airlines. He continued to amaze me with his ability to at least go through the motions of work while carrying the load of our family.

I wearily crawled back in bed, in need of physical as well as emotional rest. Where was my answer? How angry would God allow me to be with Him? The stakes were too high. I had to know before I unleashed the flood within. As I lay on my bed staring up at the ceiling, the thought came to me of Sterling, now almost two years old. If Sterling were angry with me about a decision I had made as his parent, what would I allow him to do in expressing that to me? Where were his limits? I could picture him in just a few months when his verbal skills developed—hands on his hips, intense brown eyes and thick blonde hair, chubby arms and legs, dressed in his favorite royal blue Snoopy shirt and pants, preaching to me—"Why can't I do it, Mommy? That's not fair. I don't like you."

And I had my response ready. (It's easy when you're lying on the bed imagining it, and not in the heat of the battle with these two-year-old generals!) "Sterling, I love you. That's why there are certain things you may not do. I understand that you are frustrated. But you still may not do this. And you don't have to like me, but you do have to respect and obey me as your parent. The next sixteen years will be easier for both of us if you do like me, but we'll make it either way."

I knew I would allow him to voice his anger and frustration. His limits? That he recognize that the final decision was mine as his parent. And that he respect and obey me as the final authority.

"Then God, You'll let me do that!" I had my answer. So I had my tantrum. And it was as good as any two-year-old. You know they're the experts at tantrums. The only thing missing was the volume. With sleeping grandmothers upstairs who were already concerned about us, and Mary in the family room taking care of Sterling, this had to be a quiet tantrum.

I turned over on my stomach and sobbed uncontrollably—hopefully the hardest sobs of my life. I screamed the words into my pillow, accentuating each angry word with a punch deep into the pillow. "God, I'm angry. I don't understand why it's taking so long. I don't understand why you told me that she would be a miracle and yet she continues to get worse. She almost died again yesterday. I don't understand why You don't do something about Sundays. Where do you go on Sunday? I don't understand why she went back on the respirator. You gave me a mother's heart—to love and protect this little one. What am I supposed to do with that heart while I watch Heidi suffer? Set it on the shelf? I can't watch my baby suffer any more! I don't understand what you want from me. But this is too much!"

I stopped short of voicing my ultimatum—"Either heal her or take her." That was the one boundary I was not willing to cross. As my sobbing subsided, I sat up on the side of the bed, slowly sliding my stocking feet to the mauve carpeted floor. There was silence. Not a peaceful silence. A nothing silence. God didn't strike me dead. He didn't even send lightning. Had anything changed? Well, at least my anger was out and no longer boiling within. What about God? There still seemed to be silence on His part.

I quietly emerged from our bedroom to find Grandma Boone and Sterling curled up on the sofa in the family room reading *The Poky Little Puppy.* Mary was enjoying the story, too, as she mopped the kitchen floor nearby. I will never know every person who swept the floor, washed the laundry, cleaned the kitchen, answered the phone, or played with Sterling during those months.

Another church family member Carol had brought homemade turkey noodle soup for lunch. It certainly hit the spot on that cold day. Grandma Watson had just awakened and joined Grandma Boone, Mary, Sterling, and me for lunch. Sterling kept us busy during the meal with a third of the noodles going in his mouth, a third on the high chair tray, and a third on the clean floor. The three grandmothers graciously ignored my swollen eyes and mascara-streaked cheeks. They sensed my depression and offered words of encouragement on the job I was doing as Heidi's mother. Aren't grandmothers wonderful! They've done your job before and know how challenging it can be even under the best of situations.

I spent the early afternoon hours playing with Sterling, mainly because I wanted to be with him, but partially to soothe my conscience for slipping past him that morning on our return from IHOP. We placed the colorful plastic Fisher-Price blocks into the appropriate holes in the lid of the yellow bucket. He giggled with surprise each time the round block disappeared into the round hole. Then we bundled up for a walk around the block with the red wagon.

It was one of the rare times I softened on nap schedule and allowed him to stay up until three o'clock. As we rocked and sang in his upstairs bedroom, I was again reminded of how well he seemed to be handling this family crisis. Much of the credit went to Grandma Watson and Grandpa and Grandma Boone who were spending many special bonding moments with him in Chuck's and my absence. I quietly placed a sleeping Sterling in his crib and slipped downstairs to freshen up make-up and hair before leaving for the hospital.

Miriam Watson telephoned. She and her family had just returned from Costa Rico, and she wanted an update of the past month. Wow! Where should I even start?

All I could say was, "Miriam, your prophecy was right on target. She has definitely gotten worse before getting better. And let me tell you about the last forty-eight hours!"

My anguish and questioning were obvious as I related the crisis events of Sunday and the depths that Monday had held so far.

"Vickie, I know that you and I will never understand this, but things are not as they appear in regard to Heidi suffering. God is bigger than that. She is not suffering in the way that it appears to us."

I listened quietly, taking it in. God had ministered that same word to me several nights earlier. I had wanted to believe it, but it just didn't make rational sense. How could that be? How could she not be suffering when we were watching her gasp for breath, choke on mucous, cough until she was void of strength, scream as they tried multiple IV insertions. How could she not be suffering? This must be my way of dealing with it. Pretend that she's not suffering. And yet God had just given Miriam the same word.

"You need to not go to the hospital tonight," Miriam continued. "Stay at home. Rebuild your strength physically, emotionally, and spiritually. You just need to close your door and listen to praise music. Let God minister to you. Sleep."

When Chuck arrived home a few minutes later, he had a plan. "I don't think you're supposed to go today, Vickie. You need to stay here and rest. Go to bed early tonight. I'll be okay alone."

I told him about Miriam's call. And it was obvious that I certainly had nothing to give. As we kissed good-by at the back door, he gently reminded me, "Please go to bed early and get some rest."

During the remaining hour of the afternoon, I whittled away at the ever-present stack of mail. Between the cards of encouragement and the medical bills, our mail box was crammed every day. It was a quiet afternoon. I felt nothing. Was this the calm after the storm? Or the calm in the eye of the hurricane? Or was this what it's like if God leaves you—nothingness?

Grandpa arrived home from the hospital around four-thirty with no new news regarding Heidi's condition, just more of the same. Grandma Boone headed upstairs to bed to finish her "night." Her two hours of sleep at seven o'clock that morning had not been enough. Grandma

Watson shopped at Walmart for all of us while Grandpa played with Sterling, and I set the table for dinner.

That night, as in every night of Heidi's hospital stay, a delicious hot meal was delivered to our doorstep. This time, it was from our neighbor Karen. There were many other things which were provided for us, but that one daily act supplied us with nourishment which kept our physical bodies strong. Grandpa Boone, Grandma Watson, Sterling, and I enjoyed our dinner of piping hot lasagna, garlic breadsticks, crisp green salad, and cherry cheesecake. Chuck called during dinner to give an update on Heidi. She had tested negative for RSV, although she still exhibited every symptom of a severe case of RSV. *Did it really matter that she didn't have the virus if she had every problem associated with it? She was back on the respirator, wasn't she?*

Grandma Boone's diary entry (written late that night) effectively summarized where we were medically:

> It looks like she needs (1) tricuspid valve repaired; (2) right diaphragm (unparalyzed) to start working so she can breathe easier; (3) collapsed portions of both lungs to be re-inflated with oxygen so she can breathe easier; (4) healing for the source of infection (whatever it is) that is causing coughing, temperature, vomiting and crying; (5) strengthening of her veins so they can continue with one IV and not have to keep starting another one or do surgery for another direct line in the chest . . .; (6) to be able to stay on Vickie's milk with fortifier and gain some weight . . . fast breathing is using up all her calories and she hasn't been able to gain any weight . . . slow her breathing down; (7) to get off of respirator . . . (8) Lord, take the fear out of her eyes.

On that night any one of those obstacles seemed insurmountable to me. Together—they looked like Mount Everest. And I was standing at the bottom.

Early that evening as I prepared for bed, I knew I needed God's peace to help me fall asleep. I sat on the floor beside our bed selecting a cassette tape of soft worshipful music that would hopefully minister to my weary spirit. As I dropped the tape into the Sony player, I impatiently waited for the music to begin.

Then I did my second two-year-old thing of the day. I toyed with the radio controls, waiting for the cassette tape to begin playing. Hadn't I just reprimanded Sterling for doing this last week? Still no music from the cassette. But from KVTT, a local Christian radio station, I heard the last thirty seconds of a song new to me. Tony Melendez sang—

You are His miracle, a few more steps
reach out your hand and you will see
you are His miracle, ready to be. [10]

Within a twelve-hour period God had allowed me to throw my tantrum. His response? He lovingly handed me yet another clear sign of what He was going to do in Heidi's life.

Chapter Twelve

VALENTINE'S DAY

Heidi weathered the RSV episode. Four days after going back on the respirator, she extubated herself. She had decided it was time for that tube to come out. And the doctors left it out! They took out the IVs and went back to feeding her breast milk through a stomach tube in her mouth.

Two days later they put her on nasal oxygen. She still needed help with breathing.

The next weekend, Grandma Watson returned to Ohio to her seasonal job assisting a tax accountant. She had been with us for seven weeks. But the IRS waits for no one—not even sick grandchildren!

Volunteers from our church and Chuck's office began driving Grandma Boone to the hospital at eleven o'clock each evening since it was too dangerous to be alone in that section of Fort Worth after dark. On one of those drives, a young man whose unwanted divorce had been finalized that day was able to share his pain with a willing listener. On another afternoon, Wes a dear friend from church shared with me how much he had enjoyed driving Mother to the hospital the night before. "I could listen to her talk for hours. She has the most beautiful Southern accent!"

Many people had expressed concern over the mounting financial load. We had no idea what the final tally would be but it was daily shooting upward by the thousands. Our church family and friends had generously given $6,235 to a Heidi Joy fund, to be used as needed for medical expenses. We knew that we had good insurance coverage through American Airlines, but there was a limit even to the best. And there would be voluminous paperwork ahead. But that would come later. Our focus now was Heidi—getting her well and home.

Chuck walked in from the office one afternoon and handed me a memo from American Airlines to all management employees regarding health insurance. Because of pilot arbitration resulting in an insurance change, there would also be a change in our package—"an increase in the major medical lifetime maximum for active employees from $500,000 to $1,000,000." No one was increasing coverage during those days! This was a "tighten your belt" business climate. And yet Heidi's dollar limit had just been doubled—$1,000,000! God continued to provide for *every* need in amazing ways.

After a week of struggling with only the nasal oxygen to help her breathe, Heidi had to go back on CPAP on Saturday, January 18. It had been a tough week for her with her heart rate climbing to over 200 many times and her carbon dioxide level going as high as 96 (below 45 was normal). With CPAP came the irritation of the nasal passages and a continual stream of thick mucous. In one sense breathing was easier, yet in another sense the mucous made it more difficult. It was a catch 22.

When she went back on CPAP the doctors laid out their proposal for the next steps:

(1) Surgically insert a tube directly into her stomach from the outside right at her abdomen. The g-tube (gastrointestinal) would be used for feedings directly into the stomach. Then we could take

the feeding tube out of her throat. The new tube could painless-
ly take care of feedings for an extended period of time.

(2) Do a tracheotomy—a hole in the front of her neck through which
a respirator tube could be inserted indefinitely. This would allow
her to stop working so hard at breathing, and be back on the respirator without the discomfort of the tube in her mouth.
Without the extra work of breathing, her heart could rest more
and she would hopefully grow stronger.

(3) Tack down the right paralyzed diaphragm. It had been paralyzed
for at least a month now, so there was very little chance of it ever
working. Tacking it down might help a little with her breathing,
but it would take away any opportunity for the diaphragm to
start working again.

(4) Consider the Special Care Unit—two rooms in the hospital with a
home-type setting for children who would be there for extended
periods of time.

It was five days before I even agreed to look at the Special Care Unit.
Every time the nurse brought it up, I found some excuse—just getting
ready to leave, time to pump breast milk, needed to make a phone call—
anything. We were not interested. Our daughter was not going to be here
for "an extended period of time." Two months had been far too long.

After five days of avoiding it, Nurse Sarah finally talked me into it.
"Vickie, it's in my instructions for taking care of Heidi that I'm to show
you the Special Care Unit. I'll be in trouble if I don't."

Chuck had been nudging me for days to at least be cooperative and
look at it. He had no more intentions of Heidi being there than I did.
Sarah's plea and Chuck's nudging were the only reasons I finally agreed.
We wove our way deep into the bowels of the hospital. Down corridors
hidden away behind the NICU.

As we entered the door, Sarah tried to reassure me. "It really is more of a home atmosphere than the NICU. They turn the lights off at night. The schedule is more normal with regular waking and sleeping hours. It's the closest thing to home without being there."

A nurse introduced herself and briefly explained the daily routine. "Tell me about your visiting policy," I said.

"Well, we like to keep things on a schedule here, so we have a morning and an afternoon visiting time. They're two hours each so that gives you four hours a day with your child," she explained with pride. She obviously didn't know that we were the family who had been there twenty-four hours a day.

"What about the evenings?" I asked.

"Well, I guess you could return for a short time in the evening. We don't want to mess up the children's schedule. We want everyone out of here by nine o'clock. That's lights out time."

Just like home? A schedule on which I could see my child. And seeing my child at any other time would mess up her schedule? This was not my idea of home!

I glanced around, more to please Sarah than to gain information. There were two rooms in the unit, each containing two beds, a recliner and a television. The entire outer wall of each room was windows, letting in plenty of sunshine. A solid plate of glass separated the two rooms.

In the room where we stood, an infant lay napping in a crib. The other bed was empty. Next door the room seemed a little darker. Why? There was the same plentiful supply of outdoor light. A nine-year-old boy lay on the floor. He appeared to have no control over any part of his body—muscles, speech, bodily functions. When I looked at his face and saw the anguish, I could guess the reason for the seeming darkness.

"How long has he been here?" I questioned.

"Nine years," the nurse replied. "His parents abandoned him at birth due to his problems. He is now a ward of the state."

I turned and left the room, leaving Chuck and Sarah to follow. I had seen enough. Actually more than enough. Halfway back to the NICU, Sarah with her characteristic humor tried to lighten the moment. "We lost you right at the beginning on that one, didn't we, Vickie? You were out of there when she mentioned visiting hours, right?"

"You've got that right, Sarah. My daughter is *not* going into the Special Care Unit. She is *not* going to be here for years. You can write that in your report," I ended emphatically.

With a grin she responded, "I can't say I'm surprised." We all burst into laughter. It was a good release for the tension of the moment.

We were equally unimpressed with the other three parts of the plan—the g-tube, the tracheotomy, and tacking down the diaphragm. Once again we were putting on the brakes. Trying to stand firmly yet graciously against the doctors' plan. Not that they were wrong from a medical standpoint. But we knew that it wasn't the direction God was leading us for Heidi.

One morning I sat by Heidi's bedside with my Bible propped on her bed while reading aloud. From where I sat I could easily see the entrance to the unit. A new nurse entered, glancing our way, and then moved on. By now I could guess her thoughts. "You're reading to a newborn? Don't you think you're rushing things a bit?" What would she have said had she known it was the Bible? But by now it didn't matter to me what people thought as long as we were following God's directives.

Within a minute the nurse had backtracked and came to Heidi's bedside to introduce herself. "Hi, I'm Carolyn. I've been away from here for ten years raising my children. Today is my first day back, so I just wanted to introduce myself."

"Welcome back, Carolyn. I'm Vickie and this is Heidi." I then gave her a brief history of Heidi's life.

"I noticed that you were reading the Bible to your daughter. That's great!" Carolyn said.

"We've had excellent medical care here, but it is God who has been ultimately pulling her through," I explained.

"That's interesting. I asked God to let me see a miracle when I returned to work," Carolyn said.

"Well, this is the bed to watch!" I boldly proclaimed.

After six days of fighting the CPAP, Heidi pulled the tube out at five-thirty Saturday morning. I was spending the night with her and had watched her misery for hours. Every time she moved her head, her nose bled from the irritation of the tube. When she pulled out the tube there was quite a bit of blood on the opposite end of it, indicating that the same thing was happening inside her body.

When our nurse Paula started to put the new tube into her bloody nose, I stopped her. "As a parent, I would like to request that you not put it back in."

"Well, you know we have to," she replied kindly.

"Paula, I know that as a nurse you have to follow the orders. But would you please tell the doctor that the parent has requested that you call him. I want him to look at her."

She returned in a few minutes. "I called the head nurse. We have to put this in."

"Paula, I don't want to get you in any kind of trouble. And I'll take the full responsibility for this. But as her parent I'm telling you not to put the tube back down her until we've talked to the doctor. She's already resting better in the few minutes that it's been out. And it's obvious that she has been bleeding internally from the irritation it caused."

She once again left the bedside. I couldn't believe this was me. But Heidi looked like a war zone once again. And she needed someone to stand up for her. I also knew that Dr. Smith was considering taking her off of CPAP that morning—only a few hours away.

When Paula returned, she said, "Well, we'll leave it out until Dr. Smith returns in three hours. Meanwhile we'll put her on the nasal canula (oxygen delivered at the opening of her nostrils)."

"That's great!" At the least she would get three hours of relief from the tube.

I felt that Paula possibly agreed with me, but she could have never stated it. Her job was to carry out the doctor's orders.

Heidi rested well during those few hours, the best sleep she had that week. I sat there thinking about what I had done. Chuck wasn't going to believe this one! It was totally out of character for me. What if I got us all kicked out of there? But I knew it was the right decision. God's peace confirmed it.

When Dr. Smith arrived that morning he walked immediately to Heidi and grinned. "Well, Miss Heidi, you took yourself off the respirator several weeks ago. Now I understand that you've decided to take yourself off the CPAP. You seem to be calling the shots here, little lady."

"Dr. Smith, it's my fault. I want to be sure that Paula doesn't get in trouble . . ."

He stopped me with an uplifted hand and a smile. "It's okay, Mrs. Watson. I understand. And I agree with Heidi. It *is* time to get that tube out. And we were going to take it off today anyway. She seems to be doing fine without it. You'll also be glad to know that her x-rays this morning showed that two of the three collapsed portions of her lungs are inflated. And her last carbon dioxide level was in the 40's, near normal. You know her last sonogram showed that her heart had reduced in size to almost normal. I think the reduced pressure of the heart on the lungs is affecting everything in a favorable manner."

Turning back to Heidi, he said, "Heidi, you never cease to amaze me! Just keep it up, little one!" She beamed quietly, her big brown eyes taking in every word.

"Thank you, Dr. Smith. We've been waiting a long time for a report like this. Thank you very much." I made a beeline for the phone. This news would be a fun way to start the day for those at home in Bedford! And what a delight to finally send good news across the prayer chain.

Grandma Boone spent that night with Heidi. It was a special time:

> I went in at 11:00 p.m. and Heidi Joy was getting her first tub bath by Paula. She was wide eyed and so precious. I held her for one and one-half hours, talking and singing to her. She cooed and watched me, listening intently. She moved her mouth and tried so hard to talk. I just loved it. We prayed and God gave me the blessed assurance that He is making "Something Beautiful" out of Heidi's life. This was one of the most blessed times in my whole life of fifty-nine and one-half years. God was so real and I just sat amazed in His presence with our littlest angel in my arms. Thank you, Lord, for this special visitation from you. I needed that. Oh, how I needed that.

It was now Sunday, January 26. During the month of January, we had seen Heidi make baby steps of improvement. And they were starting to add up, finally in the right direction.

On that Sunday afternoon, I gave Heidi her first bottle at nine and one-half weeks old. She took 15 cc's—1/2 ounce—in forty-five minutes. Her hair and clothing were drenched with sweat from the work of nip-pling. She burned up more energy in drinking the milk than she received from it. But we were elated. It was another step in the right direction.

The news of Heidi's bottle success spread rapidly through the unit. Crystal came racing back to her bedside when she came on duty that night. She had administered her breathing treatments many times over the past months. But her tie to our family had gone much deeper than that of respiratory therapist. This bubbly blonde in her twenties also shared the common bond of a vital Christian walk. It was she who told us later about the impact that Heidi had on both believers and non-believers among the staff.

"Those of us who were Christians had to decide how boldly we would stand. In staff meetings when Heidi's case was discussed, they always mentioned that the family wasn't accepting the facts. That they were holding on to some spiritual idea and were convinced that she would live. We had to choose whether or not to speak up and say that we understood where you were coming from. That God could heal Heidi. It was a challenge for us. She affected all of our lives here on the unit," Crystal said.

We had been able to share with Crystal the spiritual side of Heidi's journey. We had already invited her to Heidi's dedication—whenever. Like many others, she knew our family well by now. We knew her busy, fun dating life. There had been several guys just in the short time we had known her. So we had also been able to share about our marriage rela-tionship. On this Sunday afternoon, Crystal looked like a cheerleader as she came bounding back to Heidi's side.

"I heard the news. A bottle! Way to go, Heidi! That's our girl! And I can't believe I'm telling you this already, but I can't wait any longer! You know your song for Heidi?"

"Oh, yes. The one Sandi Patti sings—'You Are a Masterpiece,'" I replied.

"Yes. Vickie, I'm a singer. I wasn't going to tell you, but I've bought the sound track tape of it. I've started practicing it because I want to sing it to Heidi at her dedication. That's my gift to her. I was going to call your pastor and surprise you, but when I heard she took a bottle I couldn't wait. It's getting closer!" she beamed.

We knew she was right. Heidi had taken one-half ounce of milk from a bottle. And it was on a Sunday. Two more reasons to be grateful!

The doctors agreed to wait another week before making decisions about the g-tube, the tracheotomy, and the tacking down of the diaphragm. Meanwhile we were allowed to try bottle feeding twice a day. The majority of her milk continued to go down the feeding tube in her mouth, but this was a good start.

During that last week of January, my concern for Chuck grew. He was showing the strain of carrying a full-time job at American, a part-time job at the church, and a daughter in the hospital for ten weeks. I wasn't sure how much longer he could continue at this pace. The white hairs on his head were increasing rapidly.

When he entered the house on Friday afternoon the thirty-first, I was amazed at the weariness in his steps. We hugged and kissed. "Well, you made it through another week and another month, honey. I don't know how you're doing it apart from supernatural strength," I said.

Wordlessly he pulled a card from the pocket of his suit coat and handed it to me. It was from his employees at American.

> We have wanted to do more to lighten your load at
> this time and haven't known what else to do. But we
> have gotten special approval through Marge to work our
> days off during the month of February. You will have the
> month off to be with your family and will receive full
> pay. See you in a month!

I couldn't believe it! We stood there holding each other and weeping.
As we cried, I felt the relief flooding through Chuck's body. He was at the
end of his reserves. And God had just thrown him a rope.

"Now to Him who is able to do exceeding abundantly beyond all that
we ask or think, according to the power that works within us, to Him be
the glory . . ." (Ephesians 3:20-21, NASB) This was certainly far beyond
what we would have dreamed of or asked. Once again God's provision
was bountiful and just in time. He had never been late for us. (Although
He had certainly missed some great opportunities to be early!)

We were now into the first week of February. Sterling had turned two
years old, and Heidi was almost eleven weeks old. The doctor's report?
She is better in every way. She needs to gain three pounds and learn to
bottle feed totally before she goes home. *Did someone say **Home?***
Yes!!!!!!!!!!!!

I began spending my days at the hospital, taking over as much of
Heidi's daily routine and feedings as possible. Medications, breathing
treatments, and physical therapy to teach her how to suck on a nipple.
Babies are born with the sucking instinct. Since she had not used it in the
two and one-half months of her life, it had to be retaught.

But the biggie was always feeding. The objective was to daily increase the amount of milk taken from the bottle as we decreased the amount that went down the feeding tube. That was the remaining obstacle keeping us at the hospital.

Her heart? The size was almost normal. The tricuspid valve was still malformed and not working properly, but the doctors said that she was "compensating well." She still turned blue if she cried. But for the most part her coloring was good. She even had pink fingernail beds! They were beautiful! Heidi's carbon dioxide levels had continued their bouncing ball routine. Up, then down. Down, then up. But they seemed to stabilize by the second week of February. We were seeing normal levels on a steady basis.

On Wednesday morning the twelfth of February, Mary had come to spend the morning at the hospital with me. A loving grandmother and a faithful intercessor from day one, she was having a great time being with Heidi.

At mid-morning, the technician came in to do her weekly sonogram of Heidi's diaphragm. As she hooked up the portable sonogram machine at Heidi's bedside, I slipped over to stand behind her. Although she would never tell us the report—it had to come through the doctor after he studied it—I always peered over her shoulder. By now we could usually spot any major changes in her heart or diaphragm.

We chatted about the spring-like weather as she rubbed the cold goop on Heidi's chest. Within minutes of placing the scope on her, we saw the upward and downward motion of the left diaphragm on the small video screen. But something was different today. It certainly looked like the right side was moving. Was I seeing things? With each breath it appeared that both sides of the diaphragm were pumping up and down in perfect rhythm. I studied the technician's face. It told me nothing. Yet she was intently watching the images on the screen.

"Is that . . . do you . . . is there some movement on the right side today? Am I seeing that correctly?" I questioned, knowing that the usual response would be, "After the doctor studies it, he will give you a report."

But this time her face broke into a smile. "Where I come from, we call that a perfect diaphragm! It's working!"

"Yes! Yes! Yes!" was all I could say with tears in my eyes.

I thought Mary was going through the ceiling. "Praise God! Hallelujah! That's what we've been asking for. Jesus did that, honey!" she explained to the technician in her excited southern drawl.

I raced to the phone, elated to send another report of healing to home and the prayer chain.

The next morning Doctors Dambro, Lai, and Smith surrounded Heidi's bed to tell us the good news. There was a party-like atmosphere. We were headed home the following day! Day eighty-five! Valentine's Day! Does God have a sense of timing or what?

The staff had continually referred to Heidi as a "heart baby" when they would explain her limitations. Each time I would later whisper in her ear, "Heidi, the only sense in which you are a heart baby is that you have a heart for Jesus." So for this "heart baby" to be headed home on Valentine's Day was perfect!

It seemed as if we had waited forever for this day. In the darkest moments, we had wondered if it would ever come. And yet when they told us, we couldn't believe it was suddenly upon us. We were going to walk out of there the next day with our baby! Heidi was going home to Willow Creek Drive in Bedford!

The rest of that day, Chuck and I "roomed in" at the hospital with Heidi. Parents spend the last twenty-four hours of the child's hospitalization in a motel-type room just down the hall from the NICU. The baby stays with them, and they take over one hundred percent care of the child—medications, breathing treatments, feedings, bathing. It gives them an opportunity to care for their child with nurses only steps away for questions or emergencies.

Grandpa and Grandma Boone, Chuck, and I had been through training to learn how to do breathing treatments and CPR. We had learned how to set up the heart monitor which she would wear at all times. It looked like a large shoulder strap purse with blinking lights and wires leading to Heidi's chest. It would sound an alarm if her heart rate went too high or too low, or if she went more than twenty seconds without taking a breath. A home nurse would visit daily to check on her heart and lungs. I felt as if we were taking a part of the hospital home! But all I cared about was that we were taking Heidi Joy Watson to Bedford!

Dr. Smith looked down at Heidi with tears in his eyes, "Heidi, you know you surprised us all. You're an amazing little girl."

"Yes. You didn't do anything by the book," added Dr. Lai. "You kept us all guessing. And you gave us some frightening moments too. I'll never forget the time your heart stopped beating as your Dad and I watched on the sonogram!"

It was a special time of reminiscing about the good and the bad times over the past months. We had become close as a team, united in caring for Heidi. And there was a mutual respect. Each of us saw more clearly how the other had been used—the doctors for the physical care, our family for the spiritual and emotional care, and God for the ultimate miracle of healing.

Just before they left, Dr. Dambro walked through her concerns about Heidi's feedings. She would need twenty-four ounces of milk per day to gain weight because she burned so many extra calories in the process of taking a bottle. We were using a milk fortifier to add extra calories to her milk. We felt confident in the fact that she would eat better and continue to heal even more quickly at home.

——————— ➤➤➤ ———————

Friday, February 14, started early for our friends Stan and Denise. They had prayed and visited us many times over the past months, always bringing delicious food. Denise's Italian heritage was evident in her cooking. *Yum!*

When their clock radio came on at five o'clock that morning, the first words they heard from Steve Solomon on "Praise in the Night" were, "And Heidi Joy Watson is coming home today! Praise the Lord!"

They sat up in bed, both wide awake immediately.

"Did you hear that?" asked Stan.

"Yes, I thought someone said Heidi is coming home today," Denise answered.

"Well, was that the radio or God?" asked Stan. A call to the radio station confirmed the report for them.

Our day at the hospital began with KRLD, a large secular radio station, interviewing Chuck in the lobby. This made a great Valentine's story for them. They played the interview several times throughout the day. We later received reports of friends hearing the news in bank lobbies and on elevators. Isn't God creative!

The day was beautiful—sunshiny, crisp, and clear. But even thunderstorms would have been beautiful to me that day. All that mattered was that we would walk out of there with Heidi. She would see the sunshine. Breathe the fresh outdoor air—one hundred percent. No oxygen except that which God was supplying.

Between breathing treatments and feedings, we had been up every two hours throughout the night. But the excitement of the day wasn't dimmed by lack of sleep. The morning hours were busy—paperwork for dismissal, pharmacy instructions, heart monitor, breathing machine, setting up home nursing visits, final medical instructions, good-byes to our medical "family" of eighty-five days, taking pictures, loading the van.

It was early afternoon by the time we placed Heidi in her car seat for the first time. I sat beside her holding the heart monitor on my lap. Mother and Sterling were in the back seat. Dad was driving and Chuck rode up front with him. He was too excited to drive.

As soon as Nurse Katie closed the van door, I whispered to Dad, "Get out of here as fast as you can. I keep thinking someone's going to run out the door at the last minute yelling, 'Stop! We've made a mistake! She can't go home yet!' I won't believe it's real until I lay her in the cradle in our bedroom."

When we finally rounded the corner onto our street, home was a beautiful sight. Our front yard was filled with loving friends clapping and cheering! And there were banners! "Welcome Home." "Miracles Happen." "Praise the Lord!" "Heidi Joy Watson—Noble One of Joy." Heidi's flag was still waving atop the flagpole! And even the yellow pansies had patiently waited for this moment!

As I stepped out of the van holding Heidi close, I whispered, "You're home, Heidi. This is home. And you made it, honey." With that realization, the tears came. Wonderful tears of joy, replacing the months of painful tears.

We gathered in the front yard, surrounded by precious friends. They had stood with us faithfully for months. Now they were there to celebrate Heidi's homecoming with us. There had been many times of prayer in our home over the years. But this was the first one on the front lawn! And no one was shy. This was victory! These were prayers of thanksgiving! God had been faithful!

As we said good-bye to friends and slipped into the front door of the house, the weariness hit. But it was a good weariness. The day had been filled with milestones. I kicked off my shoes and gratefully sank into the cushions on the living room sofa with Heidi snuggled on my chest. It felt right! This was where we belonged.

Gaylene had sent Heidi a special welcome home letter which blessed us all:

> Dear Heidi Joy, there are some things I've been waiting to tell you, but since Mom and Dad and Sterling need your ears for sweet words right now, I'll just write them down and tuck them away for later.
>
> First of all, WELCOME HOME! We're so glad you're finally here. We've waited and prayed, with many others, for this day to come.
>
> Second, I want to tell you, "I love you." . . .
>
> Mostly, I wanted to tell you how the testimony of your young life and healing have strengthened my relationship with the Lord. Although my trust in the Lord has mostly grown to a "faith, and not by sight" maturity, I have been unwilling to trust Him wholeheartedly since the death of my brother. My disappointment with the circumstances of life became a disappointment with my Heavenly Father, a misdirected emotion. Since your birth, I've joined in praying for your healing, really desiring for God to prove that He could heal you. I've waited in earnest for the "good report." And praise His Name, He has been faithful. You are healed. He has heard the cries of His children and has fulfilled His promises to your family, to you, and to your offspring. As He has been Jehovah Rapha, so shall He continue to be the "I AM" in your life, in mine, and in all who place their trust in Him. All fear is gone. I trust Him again without reservation

and I pray that someday soon you'll recognize and receive with your heart the sweet Savior that you've seen standing by your bed since the beginning days of your life . . .

Welcome home, Heidi. I love you. Bless you for blessing my life.

We continued to be amazed at how God was working in the lives of so many people.

Awhile later, I headed to the recliner in our bedroom to rock Heidi to sleep. It had been a big day for her, too! Mike slipped into our bedroom with Chuck to give us a video tape. He had recorded the day for us, beginning that morning at the hospital. How appropriate that this friend who had shared in our Job Day would be the one documenting Heidi's homecoming.

As he handed me the video, tears glistened in the eyes of this intense military man. "I have one request," he said. "Not for now, but sometime later. Someday could I just sit down and hold her for a minute?"

"Oh, Mike, you can do it now," I said, placing her in his arms.

We watched in amazement as Mike's body shook with sobs. "I didn't know if this day would ever come. I've thought so many times about my challenging you to change your mind about not having children. I wondered if I had been wrong. I wondered if you wished you had never listened to me. I wondered if you regretted the decision to have children."

"Oh, no, Mike," Chuck said. "I wouldn't change a thing. I can't imagine our lives without Sterling and Heidi."

"And as hard as it has been, it has been worth it," I added. "Look at her. She's a miracle from God. And we could have missed this. No, even if we could, we would never change our decision to have children."

It was a poignant picture of how deeply our pain had been carried by our friends. Minutes later, there was another reminder. As I laid a sleeping Heidi in her cradle for the first time, cousin Jessica slipped into our bedroom and curled her arm around my neck as I knelt by the cradle.

"She's home, Jessica. Thank you for praying," I whispered.

"So is she not going to die, Aunt Vickie?" she gently questioned.

"No, Jessica, she's not going to die. She is going to be just fine."

It had been an unbelievably long journey for the adults. What must it have been for a six-year-old prayer warrior?

And now every February 14, we celebrate Heidi Home Day in our family. We string heart garlands across the dining room and fill the center of the table with teddy bears holding hearts. We devour a heart-shaped chocolate sour cream cake decorated with white icing and chocolate kisses. And we walk through the story of God's faithfulness in healing Heidi and bringing her home.

That's why everyone puts up all those hearts, isn't it!

Chapter 13

Jesus Hold Me

Nine days later on Sunday, February 23, Heidi was dedicated to the Lord.

What a moment of triumph when I finally dressed her in the beautiful white christening gown I had longingly gazed at for almost three months. From the first note of the opening song, I knew we weren't the only ones there to party. The praise was jubilant! We had finally won one as a church body and we celebrated!

The theme for the day—To God Be the Glory! The service ended with the worship team singing Andraé Crouch's song "My Tribute." As I stood cradling Heidi in my arms, the words ministered powerfully to me. I had heard these words sung every way possible over the years, but today the meaning and the gratitude were deeper than ever before. "With His blood He has saved me, With His power He has raised me, To God be the glory for the things He has done."[11] That summarized the day perfectly. That's what the party was all about!

We spent the next weeks feeding Heidi—literally. It took one hour to get one ounce of milk down. And she needed to drink twenty-four ounces during each twenty-four hour period.

After two and one-half weeks, she was losing weight and on the edge of dehydration, so back to the hospital we went. It was a jolt! I couldn't believe we were there again. Six days later, we came home with a feeding tube down her nose, seven medications, and one frustrated mother.

Her care had been intense before, but now it took Chuck, Grandpa and Grandma Boone, and me twenty-four hours a day to care for her. We fed her every three hours around the clock. And we had to hold her upright for an hour after each feeding because so much of the milk came right back up the tube.

We documented feeding amounts and times, throw-up amounts, heart monitor alarms, breathing treatments, twenty-three doses of medicine—there was never a spare moment. We divided the night in half with Chuck and me on the first half, and my parents on the second half. A two-hour span of uninterrupted sleep became a cause for praise.

Chuck had returned to work by now. In the back of my mind, I knew the day would come when Dad and Mother would have to go home. They had been with us since November except for a one-week span at home after Heidi's dedication. Although we would have loved it (and had begged them to move here), I knew they couldn't be here forever.

One afternoon one of our encouragers called and asked if I had seen an interview on the Christian television channel that morning. It had reminded her of Heidi. I responded as calmly as possible, "No, we haven't had time to watch TV. Heidi's care keeps us pretty busy."

"Oh, I know that. I'm just talking about when you catch fifteen minutes of TV here or there throughout your day," she responded.

I ended the conversation quickly and stood in the kitchen shaking my head with wonder at Mother. "Do you know what she wanted? She wanted to know if I had seen something on TV! I wanted to tell her that I brushed my teeth at nine o'clock last night for the first time that day. And it wasn't because I have a hygiene problem!"

I thought Mother was going to pick up the phone and call her. You know how we mothers are when it comes to our children! This gave me a new appreciation for parents with high-need children. There were many people who had done this for years! And I had no idea of the load with which they had been living.

A week later, Chuck and I met in the kitchen at midnight, getting a drink of water. We had been trying to protect his sleep as much as possible because of his work schedule. As we chatted for a few minutes seated at the kitchen table, I realized that this was the more difficult time for the two of us. There was very little time together. We met over a feeding tube at Heidi's bedside or studying a feeding schedule to see where we were on the twenty-four hour quota of milk. There seemed to be no time for each other.

All four of us adults had been equally wiped out after dinner that evening so the dishes were still in the sink. As I started loading the dishwasher, Chuck came to my side and put his arms around me. "You've got to get sleep, Vickie. The kitchen can wait."

"But I don't know that it's ever going to be any better, so I've got to figure out how to do all of this," I cried, pouring out the thoughts that had been on my mind for days. "Sooner or later Mother and Dad will have to go home, and you've got to have enough rest to function at work. So it's up to me to figure out how to do everything. I just didn't think God would send us home with a sick baby."

There it was—the core of my disappointment since Heidi had come home this second time. I thought the hard part was over. But I was realizing that we had brought home a baby who needed a very high level of care.

But Heidi did continue to improve over the months ahead—slowly but surely. The feeding tube came out, and the medications were dropped one by one. By her first birthday, she was medication free—a major milestone!

We had a special birthday invitation printed for her party. On the cover was a picture taken during the first few days of her life—tubes and all. In vivid contrast at its side was another photo taken nine months later of an animated little girl sitting up with big smiling eyes, curly hair and the caption "Miracle Heidi." The inside carried this message:

THANK YOU

You prayed steadfastly
You blessed us with generous gifts
You brought delicious meals

You prayed earnestly
You sent words of encouragement
arriving at just the right moment
You gave Chuck a much-needed leave from work

You prayed fervently
You decorated our home for Christmas
You answered our phone

You surrounded us with love and prayer
You gave Sterling a birthday party
You cleaned our house

You prayed unceasingly
You drove family members to the hospital
You lovingly cared for both Heidi and Sterling

You stood with us, still believing and praying
And God Sent the Miracle!

"I shall not die, but live, And tell of the works of the Lord."
Psalm 118:17 (NASB)

We then gave an update on Heidi:

Today we are enjoying a delightful one-year-old who is exploring every inch of her world—pulling up, crawling, climbing, whatever it takes to get there! Last week this 17-1/2 pound bundle of energy climbed a flight of stairs. Heidi is medication free. Her pulmonologist released her this month with these words—"She's a normal child lung-wise." Her cardiologist reports that her heart is normal in size. The tricuspid valve leakage is significantly less. Heidi readily takes bottles from us and will eat anything *she* can put into her mouth. She's a woman who knows what she wants! Developmentally she is right on schedule. In spite of all she has been through, Heidi is a joyful child and daily reminds us of God's mercy and power. To God be the glory!

CELEBRATE WITH US!! On November 21, 1992, Heidi will be one-year-old. For her birthday, she would appreciate a letter from you sharing your part of her story. We want Heidi to know the full story of her miracle from family, friends, and medical team. We want her to know how God used you to care for her family and for her during this year, and we only have a small piece of the puzzle. Please help us in telling Heidi her story.

When: Saturday, November 21, 1992

Drop-in 2:00-4:00 p.m.

Where: Our home, 3825 Willow Creek Drive
              Bedford, Texas

The letters poured in from all over the country. Many shared that her picture had been on their refrigerator doors over the past year as their families had daily prayed for her. Some still keep the "before and after" one year announcement pictures posted in their homes as an encouragement for miracles in their lives today.

The people also poured in to our home that Saturday afternoon—around two hundred visited. Several of her NICU nurses called that day with congratulations. What a celebration of God's faithfulness!

Late that night I wrote in my journal for the first time since that painful day in early December when I had stopped writing. It had been almost a year. This time it was a letter to Heidi—the beginning of what I wanted her to know about the miracle of her life:

November 21, 1992
Dear Heidi,

   It's midnight—the ending of your first birthday—and the ending of your first year. You were beautiful today, Heidi. So full of life and joy. You knew it was a special day from the moment you awakened this morning. You stood alone for the first time. And the way you sat on our bathroom vanity, playing with my earrings while Grandma Boone and I dressed you. You knew you were the party girl—dressed in your soft burgundy dress with the lacy bows and the cross-stitched "Miracle Heidi" collar. Grandma made it especially for this day.

   You put on quite a show for the newspaper photographer also. And you watched the festivities, playing with the balloons and ribbons, so full of life and joy. You took your first steps at your birthday party. What timing! Jesus and you had been waiting for that moment.

Then tonight you couldn't go to bed. At 9:00 you were still giggling and joyfully celebrating downstairs in our bedroom. You took a few more steps, played peek-a-boo, and continued to stand on your own and giggle at yourself. My word picture of you today is summed up with one word — JOY. It is all over you. You are such a delight.

Today I've made myself focus on this day and the celebration of what I see now. I'm frightened to look too closely at a year ago on this date. Frightened that if I look for a moment too long, the tears will start and the pain will come back.

I just finished reading your birthday cards and letters. The tears started with those, so I guess it's okay to peak just a little bit closer.

Your Daddy and I had left the house at 5:00 a.m. that Thursday morning for the hospital to welcome you into the world . . .

What a special day Jesus gave us on that Saturday. What a beautiful reminder of His faithfulness to us as a family. And the letters spilled out of our mailbox for days, arriving from eighteen states as well as France, England, Sri Lanka, and New Guinea. It was an eye-opening picture of how steadfast and wide-spread the prayers had been. We were amazed to hear what God had done in the lives of others.

It was a blessing to our family when our children

actually saw God answer their prayers. Your story also touched another family who was praying for their unborn child who had been diagnosed with three mysterious cysts on his brain. Many prayers and six weeks later, the cysts are gone. Your story brought them hope! Randal & Andi

. . . Your Dad and I laid hands on you and prayed. This was the beginning of what was to be a very special time in my life as Jesus *used your circumstance for my growth.* . . . We *are* our brother's keeper. We *do* have a place in each other's lives. Many of us learned things about ourselves that would not have been learned had it not been for Heidi Watson . . . While God was "remodeling" your little body, He was doing major renovation on many people in the church. I saw you as a "small" picture of the greater story. Each person had a job. Each person had a responsibility. Gary

We all learned a lot through you. We learned how precious life is—especially little helpless babies. We learned how to really pray for others, and how to trust God. We learned as a church how to be united in one cause or mind for someone in need—that was you and your family. People fasted . . . and prayed around the clock for you, baked meals for your family, visited you— we did what God told us to do as a part of His church. But I think most of all we learned to really trust God— even when we wanted to give up and lose faith and think that you wouldn't make it. Through this we learned (especially your mom and dad) that God is faithful. . . . We all learned that God's Word is true. Ken & Cheryle

. . . I'll have to be honest—when I made your dedication gown, I *really* couldn't believe that God asked me to do it! Because I wasn't as sure as your momma and daddy that you were gonna make it. Thank goodness though, that I was obedient! . . . Todd & Connie

I was one of your nurses in the hospital during your first months. I'm actually one of the nurse managers there so didn't get to do very much hands-on care for you. I had more opportunity to talk to your parents and to help others who were helping you. Sometimes we nurses get too attached and too technical to see the "big picture." But I wanted you to know that we think you have turned into a beautiful little girl with a tremendous special gift—life itself. There were many times we thought we would lose you and maybe we were often too negative to you and those around you, but we had never seen any baby with your problems make it. We also saw that you had *many*, *many* special people that were so in love with you that we were trying to prepare them in case you were taken to be with the Lord. It was a difficult position for us all. But look at you now— Wow! . . . Carol

We had asked Jesus for something special for our anniversary. It's February 14. Jesus let you come home on that day. Our whole being rejoiced when your Grandpa drove the van around the corner. What a day. Jim & Mary

The first Sunday at church, a group of people gathered around Uncle Bryan and me to pray for you. I lost control and began weeping again for all the emotional and physical pain your family and you were under. Then in my prayers, I saw a very petite, 3-year-old little girl running all over the church. She was W I R E D ! It was you. You were healthy, whole and a bundle of LIFE. That was what I needed. I knew you were going to be okay. I did question that at times, and wonder why God was doing things like He was, but He had it all under control . . . I'm grateful that I was able to witness a miracle in watching you. I had never had that experience before, and had begun to wonder if it really happened in the 1990's . . . Auntie Rose

At the time I am writing this to you, I have cancer. It's called lymphoma. The doctors believe it's incurable. Sometimes when I'm feeling a little down, I remember you and your family. Those thoughts lift my spirits. So even though we haven't officially met yet, I feel like I know you because of the joy and encouragement you have already shared with me! Stephen

Stephen has stayed in our home to visit Heidi as an encouragement for his own illness. After various types of treatment, he is still fighting and winning the cancer battle four years later.

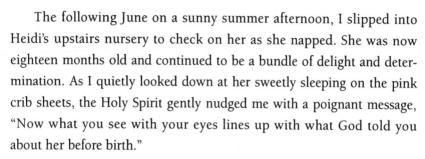

The following June on a sunny summer afternoon, I slipped into Heidi's upstairs nursery to check on her as she napped. She was now eighteen months old and continued to be a bundle of delight and determination. As I quietly looked down at her sweetly sleeping on the pink crib sheets, the Holy Spirit gently nudged me with a poignant message, "Now what you see with your eyes lines up with what God told you about her before birth."

Did it ever! The rhythmic breathing, the pink coloring, the peaceful countenance as she slept—what a beautiful picture of health! What a masterpiece!

In February following her second birthday, she came off of the heart monitor. Medication and machine free at last! By early fall Heidi was chattering away. She danced and sang her way through most days. Life was a party for her. She didn't want to miss a minute of it.

One fall Sunday morning Chuck and Heidi were enjoying an early breakfast of Cheerios together before Sterling and I awakened. She had blessed the meal with her usual, "Jesus, sank oo food, amen." After praying she continued to sit quietly with her eyes closed for a minute. That's a long time for a two and one-half year old!

Sensing the tenderness of the moment, Chuck watched her for a few minutes and then ventured a question. "Heidi, do you remember when you were a baby and sick in the hospital?"

A quiet nod was her only reply.

"What do you remember about being in the hospital?"

Her big brown eyes calmly gazed at Chuck as she replied, "Jesus hold me."

Chapter Fourteen

What Did I Learn?

Am I a different person today? Thank God, yes. What a tragedy it would be to walk through the crisis and exit unchanged!

When I look back over that first year of Heidi's life, I see that *every* single need in *every* area of our lives for *every* member of our family was bountifully supplied. Had it been painful and difficult? Yes! But had God shown Himself faithful and mighty? *Yes!* He had brought us through. More than that, He had brought us through triumphantly—better than we were before.

How am I different today? How am I hopefully better?

Oh, some ways are humorous. There was the first time Chuck and I were able to leave Heidi and Sterling overnight so we could have time alone. We drove to the quaint East Texas town of Fredericksburg for two days and one night. Our cozy cottage at the bed and breakfast was perfect. Surrounded by large magnolia trees and a white picket fence, we felt as if we had stepped back in time. Eleven hours of uninterrupted sleep . . . strolling the quiet downtown streets hand in hand . . . exploring antique shops . . . sipping limeades at the drugstore counter—it was exactly what we needed.

That evening we enjoyed a peaceful gourmet dinner back at the bed and breakfast. I felt as if we had been transported to a southern planta-tion. The high-ceilinged dining room looked out onto a magnolia lined lawn where squirrels scampered from tree to tree. Soft classical music filled the air. A single candle lit our white linen draped table for two. We were the only early diners that evening. The feedings and monitors and medications seemed worlds away as we quietly talked our way through each course of the meal.

Between courses we held hands across the table, savoring the intimate moments of quiet conversation. The scene was interrupted by a loud beeping sound coming from the next room. Within seconds we were on our feet ready to see what had caused Heidi's heart monitor to alarm. The waiter looked at us curiously as he explained that the microwave beeps when it stops. It was several years before we stopped sprinting into action on cue. We were better trained than Pavlov's dogs!

And there are still the moments when I see tears silently roll down Chuck's cheeks at the sound of a tiny infant crying on an airplane or in a meeting. Tears of memories. Of not being able to hear Heidi's cries that first month of life. Often he goes to the embarrassed new parents with words of encouragement. "Don't you worry about what others think or say. Be grateful for the sound of that baby crying. It's beautiful. It's a sign of life and health."

I married a man with a capacity for many human relationships—more than anyone I have ever known. Little did I know how that would be used in God's provision for us in time of crisis.

My first glimpse of how many friends Chuck Watson had came as we were planning our wedding. I had requested his list of names for the wedding invitation list. I waited and waited and waited. This was not like him to be this late. Each time I asked about it, he responded, "I'm working on it. It's almost done."

After several weeks he showed up at my door one night proudly bearing the finished product—a computer print-out of 1,100 family units! My image of a nice church wedding was fading away. This man was planning a convention, not a wedding!

As calmly as possible, I questioned him, "Is there any way you could at least cut the list in half? Maybe you could invite the closest of your friends instead of everyone you know?"

He assured me that these were people he considered close, but that he would do his best to shorten the list. We added my friends to the computer, and he promised to work at bringing back a shorter slate.

A week later, he brought the new print-out over, apologetic and yet proud that he had shortened it to seven hundred family units. "That includes both of our lists so I really did cut out lots of names. But this was a painful process for me," he explained. I still could not imagine anyone having that many people so close to them, but I was starting to get a clearer picture of the volume of people in this man's life.

Several days later as I worked my way through the list of names, I noticed that he had marked through the name "Mrs. Chester Austin." This was interesting.

I called him and questioned him about it. "Vickie, I know you teased me about not even knowing who some of those people were since there were so many names. I must admit that you caught me on that one. I do know her, but I admit that I couldn't remember who she was. So you will see that I did mark her off."

"Honey, Mrs. Chester Austin is my grandmother!"

It became a precious story to me of who this wonderful man Chuck really was. There were five hundred people at the wedding and fifty in the wedding party, and that was only the beginning of a life filled with wonderful friends.

And yet as I looked back over the many people who ministered to us throughout Heidi's illness, I understood that we were receiving from many whom we had been able to give to in ministry or friendship.

Our friend Ken summed it up best in a letter to us following Heidi's second hospital stay:

> . . . Even if you're discouraged or tired or worn out through all the heartache and trials you've been through the past few months—you must feel blessed and fortunate. Yes, you are very blessed. You see, behind those countless hours of praying, sleeplessness, even worry, there have been more friends and even acquaintances who have and are praying for you and Heidi.
>
> Over the years you have touched hundreds, probably thousands of lives, and they have been lifting you up to the Father in time of need. You have sowed into scores of lives, and have reaped the blessing through your little girl . . .

Do we sow into friendships and ministry for the purpose of receiving? No. But we were able to see the sowing and reaping principle at work in our situation. We had not given in order to receive. But we found ourselves reaping an abundance of blessings from these precious people who God had brought into our lives over the years.

What else did I learn about God and His plan for meeting our needs in times like this? The lessons from His classroom were life-changing for me.

I learned that God does still work miracles today—but in His timing and His way. No, we are not to demand of Him. But, yes, we are to hold on to His promises tenaciously. I am a grateful mother, awed by the power and love of God. I have purposefully shared with you the dark corridors of our journey in detail. Not to dwell on the negative. But to clearly show that this was not a neat one-two-three packaged miracle. To some (and to us) it may seem like an unbearably long journey. To others it's brief in comparison with your trek of faith.

Our story may have seemed like a nicely packaged deal as you read it, but it didn't feel that way as we walked it. Many times we felt that life was out of control. The fact that we did not see His hand working in the situation (with our limited vision) was not a true measurement of His presence. Our feelings were never an accurate yard stick for measuring His involvement. Only the Word of God is truth. And God continued to work in spite of our feelings.

I learned how the body of Christ is to work in caring for those in crisis. It was as if we were listening to the London Philharmonic Orchestra. Each instrument was finely tuned and skillfully executing its part. We didn't need an orchestra of all drums. Or all violins. Or all trumpets. We needed a mixture, with each harmoniously blending its part with the others.

That's what we received. A hot meal on our table every evening. That alone represented many people over a three-month period. Several years later, Julie apologized to me for bringing only one meal during that time. "I wanted to do more," she confessed, "but my husband was out of work at the time, and it was all that we could afford."

"Julie, do you know what I remember about the meal you sent?" I asked, deeply moved at her sacrifice. "You left a card of encouragement on the table, and I read it at 2:00 a.m. as we finished your food after a particularly difficult night at the hospital. It was exactly what I needed at that moment. And we never went without a meal. God's plan was for you to bring that one meal. That was your part. He wasn't asking you to do anything else. You owe me no apology."

What a reminder to me of the sacrifice that went into many of those meals. I now jump at the opportunity to return that blessing of a meal to other families in crisis. And I often send along a note of encouragement.

There were the lunches packed for the hospital by our neighbors and Chuck's co-workers. They went far beyond the peanut butter and jelly menu, although that would have been fine. I learned to give my creative best and to ask God what would minister in that situation. Yes, He even cares about menus!

There were telephones answered and over fifty messages a day skillfully relayed for us. What a blessing. These people showed us clearly about working within your gifting. If you can't take down a phone number or message, then God isn't calling you to that area. You are doing it out of guilt or "oughtness" and that isn't from Him. When you operate within your gifting, it is a natural outflow. It's usually what comes easily for you.

There were the specific unusual offers of help, tailor-made for our needs. Jackie wrote stacks of gracious thank-you notes. One of our church's care groups decorated our home for Christmas. Another provided Sterling's two-year-old birthday party—everything from invitations to decorations to food. Another cleaned our house. Randy (owner of a local print shop) printed five hundred copies of a birth announcement/prayer request mailing at no cost. Dorian prepared the photos and layout, also at no cost.

Those creative offers continued even after Heidi came home from the hospital. Mark called one morning to say he would be over to mow our lawn that afternoon. Carol arrived every Monday morning for months (until she moved out of state) and took our piles of dirty laundry, returning that afternoon with crisp ironed shirts and stacks of neatly folded clothes. She later told me that the reason she did it at her home was to give us back the privacy of our home.

There was Barbara who came over many weekends to take Sterling for walks or rock Heidi. There were other mothers who included Sterling in outings with their toddlers—the zoo, the park, McDonalds—fun times graciously supplied when we could not give them. There were Jill and Marianna from the baby-sitting co-op, busy mothers of four young children each, who took turns keeping Sterling one day a week for months.

These were people who simply said, "I would like to do this for you." Had they said to me, "Give me a call if you need something," it would have gone unheeded. Much of the time, I didn't even know what the logistical needs were, and I'm not sure I could have picked up the phone to ask for help. God was directing their offers.

One of the most unusual times of ministry to me was on a Sunday afternoon between Heidi's two hospital stays. A twenty-four hour prayer vigil had gone on in our living room throughout the night and day for Heidi to drink adequate milk to avoid dehydration. As they prayed, they watched her on closed-circuit television hooked into our bedroom (thanks to electronic genius Carl) to protect her from exposure to infections. It's humbling when people tell you months later that they watched you sleeping in the recliner during the night on TV!

By Sunday afternoon, Heidi still was not eating well, and my patience was gone. I couldn't spend another hour in that blue recliner trying to get one more ounce of milk down her. I tearfully handed her to Mother and escaped to an upstairs bedroom. Minutes later, Pam and Chris gently knocked on the door and entered.

Pam shared the story in her birthday letter to Heidi:

> You were not eating well. You were not very active. Your Mommy was very tired both physically and emotionally; probably spiritually as well . . . Your Daddy

came to Chris and me and asked us to please go up and talk to your Mommy and pray with her.

We were with her for at least an hour, talking to her and letting her express her feelings—including her doubts about God. He is so amazing; He wants us to be totally honest with Him, even if it means we are mad at Him or aren't sure we can trust Him . . .

Chris and I prayed with your Mommy, read lots of Scriptures (especially Psalm 23), and gave her a back rub. We could feel the peace of God enter the room as the presence of the Holy Spirit came in a powerful way.

Your Mommy was able to relax in the arms of her loving Savior, Jesus, and let Him carry her heartache and burdens for awhile.

What do I remember about that hour? I recall lying on the bed, tears streaming down my face, as Pam read Psalm after Psalm in her dramatic way that makes each verse come alive as if it were written for you alone. My knotted muscles slowly relaxed under Chris' skillful touch. My spirit and body needed peace and renewal, and that's what God supplied through these precious women operating under the Spirit's direction. God is creative and thorough in meeting our needs if we will follow His direction rather than our preconceived ideas of ministry.

Several hours later, when I returned to our bedroom to start on the next ounce of milk, I found a sleeping Heidi and a note from Mother beside the blue recliner—"Vic, you are the reason we still have Heidi. You're a super mom and don't let the Devil tell you otherwise. You're doing what's best for Heidi, and that's what mothers are for. I'm proud of you, honey. I love you. Mother." Both Heidi and I were calmer and more successful with that next feeding.

Then there were those who tucked checks in with their cards, or left them on the kitchen table as they passed through our home. And many gave to the Heidi Joy Watson fund at our church. At the end of one year, every medical bill had been paid. What a provision from God!

What a contrast to the man who stood in our entryway late one night saying, "I see no road but bankruptcy ahead for you and Chuck with the staggering medical costs. And they're still mounting, you know."

"Oh, no," I had replied. "God is not going to heal Heidi and leave us bankrupt. He's not saying, 'I can take care of her body but I can't do anything about your finances.' I don't know how we'll get there, but the money will be taken care of. There will be enough."

There were Chuck's co-workers who sacrificed their days off during February to work in his place. They will never know what a difference that made to a weary father whose stamina was gone. As I look at it now, I see clearly that they were playing their instruments within the orchestra. Doing what they could do and what no one else could.

There were the hundreds of cards we received. Prior to this, I was never a "card" person. You read them, think "oh how nice," and pitch them in the trash. But this time, I devoured the cards in our daily mail. Several years later, as I took the time to sift back through the notes and cards, reminiscing about the precious people represented in those stacks, I saw an amazing trend. Many of the cards with powerful injections of hope were from those who had walked through deep waters. I saw weekly cards from Don and Mary, our brother and sister-in-law in Ohio, who had lost their first child at birth and had spent the first month of their second child Elizabeth's life in the hospital. I had no idea of the depth of their pain when they had walked those paths. But they certainly knew where we were with Heidi. Mary's heart was in those cards. They understood how to journey alongside us, though separated by hundreds of miles.

I remember the times when I was weary with the battle. My recurring thought was, *If I'm her mother and I'm tired of praying, then others must have given up a long time ago.* One of those times, I received a call from twelve of my uncles and aunts who had gathered for a Saturday afternoon of fellowship. They each spoke no more than thirty seconds, but the encouragement sent across the phone wires from Mississippi was a powerful reminder that we were not forgotten.

Another of those times, I opened a card from a Sunday School class at a local Church of Christ bearing sixty-six names. We knew one American Airlines employee out of that group, but here were sixty-six people who said they were praying for our daughter!

Another time a card arrived from a ladies' retreat where I had spoken the previous year. They were gathered for their annual retreat and had prayed especially for us that weekend. Does a name on a card mean much? Prior to Heidi's birth, I would have said, "No." Today I would say a resounding, **"Yes."**

There were the faithful prayer warriors who stood and stood for months and months. There were those who fasted. Pastor Jim was a dynamic cheerleader encouraging the people to be steadfast in prayer. Pastor Travis was a gentle shepherd who walked the darkest paths with us. Miriam was a prophet who boldly proclaimed God's word. Pat was a faithful intercessor who travailed for Heidi.

The list goes on and on. Each person did his share, and our needs were abundantly met. No one person could have carried that overwhelming load. God didn't intend for any one person to do that. Often we think it's up to us to meet every need when we are really called to ask God what our part is in the whole picture. Which instrument we need to play within the orchestra. Each member is significant for his contribution—none more important than the other—yet each working together to create beautiful harmony.

The rewards for obedience? They are the same, regardless of the instrument played. David stated it clearly in I Samuel 30:22-24 upon returning from battle. His grumbling warriors complained, "'Because they did not go with us, we will not give them any of the spoil that we have recovered' . . . Then David said, 'You must not do so, my brothers, with what the Lord has given us, who has kept us and delivered into our hand the band that came against us . . . For as his share is who goes down to the battle, so shall his share be who stays by the baggage; they shall share alike.'" (NASB)

I pray more quickly "on the spot" today. Whether that be in a crowded room, a quiet car, or a telephone conversation. When a painful need is shared, there is much power and comfort in an arm around the shoulder and an immediate prayer. The promises for future intercession are good, but the present prayer is a great way to start that intercession.

I learned that we too often take on the needs and provisions of others beyond what God has asked. He alone has the whole picture. We are only called to do our part.

There were several times during Heidi's hospital stay that one of our parents would need to return to Ohio or Mississippi for several days to handle business matters. It was very difficult for them to pull away, and yet financial matters had to be cared for. At those times, they repeatedly apologized for leaving for even two days. And yet God had given me such a peace about His provision.

"It's okay," I repeatedly said.

"But who will stay at the hospital. And who will help with Sterling?"

"I don't know. But I know you need to take care of these business matters. So it means that God has another provision for us here. He will provide. You'll see when you return," I assured them.

And He always did provide. Too often our error isn't in obeying His prompting to help. It's in knowing our part—where it starts and where it ends. He does not call us to minister at the detriment of our own health or families. When our limits are reached, unless He supplies strength supernaturally, then we are to stop. He has another provision at that point. **He** is the provider. Not us. We are simply the instruments. Know when to start playing, but also know where the rests are within the music.

———— ➤ ————

Involve your children in intercession. Some of the most poignant cards and prayers were from young children.

Marianna wrote a letter of encouragement when Heidi was six weeks old.

> Even though I haven't talked to you or come to the hospital, our family has been praying for Heidi Joy since the day after she was born. She is really a big part of our life. We pray for her at least four times a day—at meals and bedtime. The children *never* forget to pray for her. Their prayers and faith are so wonderful. They have such faith and total trust in God. Kara (four) and Lauren (three) have named their dolls "Heidi Joy."

This past year our family had the opportunity to be a part of baby Jason's prayer support throughout several heart surgeries and eating difficulties of his first year of life. It was especially poignant to hear Heidi pray at meals, "Jesus, help Baby Jason drink his bottle." And what joy for our entire family to celebrate with Jerry and Michelle at Jason's one-year-old birthday party.

We rob our children of an early understanding of God's miracle-working power and everyday involvement in our lives because we are afraid of disappointment. God can handle His own press. At an early age, they need to experience the "yes" and "no" answers to prayer. Whether it be praying for a sick baby or to find new jeans at a good price, God wants to be involved in our daily walk. Let them hear you ask Jesus to help you find their missing pair of shoes or the crying baby's misplaced pacifier. Minutes later their "yahoo—yea Jesus" will be ample reward.

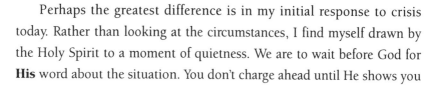

Perhaps the greatest difference is in my initial response to crisis today. Rather than looking at the circumstances, I find myself drawn by the Holy Spirit to a moment of quietness. We are to wait before God for **His** word about the situation. You don't charge ahead until He shows you or someone else His plan.

And the battle plan is different for each war. Oh, there are similarities, but He is a creative God in battle as in everything else. The Old Testament reflects many different battle plans used by God.

Once you know His plan—when you are sure that you have heard from Him and can clearly see that He backs up that plan with His Word—then you are ready to face the crisis with Him at your side.

And remember there are moments when we miss it. I'll never forget the lesson of the "On Stage—Heidi" sign. Our job is not to interpret the message, it's to walk in obedience in the battle with our eyes and ears constantly tuned to His frequency. He is our focus. He is the general who gives the orders. We are the infantry. Hang on to what He has said about the situation until the circumstances line up with what He has told you. It may be an hour or days or months or years. But "your faith should not stand in the wisdom of men, but in the power of God." (I Corinthians 2:5, KJV)

Epilogue

Twenty-eight months after Heidi's birth, God blessed us with Holly, a sweet, healthy little girl. The early days of nurturing and holding that had been painfully stolen with Heidi were graciously restored with Holly. It was a healing process for me and a triumph for our family as we brought home a healthy newborn on the second day of her life. And twenty-four months after Holly we welcomed Landon into our family—a healthy ten-pound two-ounce boy. We're grateful that we didn't miss the blessing of Holly and Landon out of fear. God does restore what the enemy has stolen. Our household is never boring these days with Sterling (6), Heidi (4), Holly (2), and Landon (6 months)—truly blessings from the Lord.

Heidi's dark hair has now lightened to golden blonde curls. And those saucer-like brown eyes don't miss a thing as she skips and sings her way through each day. Life is a party, and she lives each moment to the fullest. On a recent sunshiny morning as we headed out the back door to run errands, Heidi waved her arms in the air and skipped her way to the garage chiming out, "Good morning, birds!" She is a precious reminder to us to find delight in each day.

At her annual cardiology check-up this year, Dr. Lai beamed as he knelt at Heidi's side with her arm linked around his neck while she sang "Jesus Loves Me."

Her heart? It's fine. Restrictions on Heidi? She will take an antibiotic prior to dental work or surgery as a precaution against infection in the heart. Other restrictions? None.

Dr. Smith's words in a letter to our insurance company in June of 1992 sum it up best:

> Heidi had a long, difficult and very complicated hospital course . . . Considering the seriousness of Heidi's medical problems, the fact that she is home with her family, growing and developing normally, is nothing short of miraculous.

The calling on Heidi's life: "I shall not die, but live, and declare the works of the Lord." (Psalm 118:17, KJV)

October 1, 1996
Bedford, Texas

NOTES

1. "Masterpiece" by Brent Alan Henderson, Craig Patty, Michael Patty, Gloria Gaither. Copyright © 1989 Steadfast Music/Knotty Pine Music (administered by Addison Music Co.)/Sandi's Songs Music (administered by Addison Music Co.)/Gaither Music Co. (administered by Gaither Copyright Management). Used by permission.

2. Source of medical book unknown. Provided by medical personnel.

3. "Rejoice For The Steps" by Henry Gaskins © 1989 Integrity's Hosanna! Music/ASCAP. All rights reserved. Used by permission.

4. "Emmanuel" Words and Music: Bob McGee, 1976. Copyright 1976 C.A. Music (div. of Christian Artists Corp.) All rights reserved. ASCAP.

5. "For Those Tears I Died" by Marsha J. and Russ Stevens. 1969 Bud John Songs, Inc. (ASCAP). Administered by EMI Christian Music Publishing.

6. "He Is Able" Words by Rory Noland, Music by Greg Ferguson and Rory Noland. © 1988 Maranatha! Music (Administered by The Copyright Company, Nashville, TN). International copyright secured. All rights reserved. Used by permission.

7. From *A Woman's Guide to Spiritual Warfare* © 1991 by Quin Sherrer and Ruthanne Garlock. Published by Servant Publications, Box 8617, Ann Arbor, Michigan 48107. Used with permission.

8. "He Who Began A Good Work in You" Words and Music by Jon Mohr. © 1987 Birdwing Music/Jonathan Mark Music (ASCAP). All rights reserved. Administered by EMI Christian Music Publishing and Gaither Copyright Management.

9. This material is taken from *My Utmost for His Highest* by Oswald Chambers, page 356. Copyright © 1935 by Dodd Mead & Co., renewed © 1963 by the Oswald Chambers Publications Association, Ltd.., and is used by permission of Discovery House Publishers, Box 3566, Grand Rapids, MI 49501. All rights reserved.

10. "You Are His Miracle" Words & Music by Doug Eltzroth. Copyright © 1989 Shepherd's Fold Music (BMI). Administered by EMI Christian Music Publishing. All rights reserved. Used by permission.

11. "My Tribute" by Andraé Crouch. 1971 Bud John Songs, Inc. (ASCAP). Administered by EMI Christian Music Publishing.

For additional copies of

Miracle Heidi:
When Doctors Couldn't . . . God Could

contact:

STERLING PRESS INTERNATIONAL
Post Office Box 415
Bedford, Texas 76095
817 318-7900

Send $12.99 + $2.00 shipping and handling
(total $14.99) for each book ordered. Check or
money order accepted. Deliveries outside of
the continental U.S.A. require additional
shipping charge.